GW00499464

THE NEWBORN
IN THE INTENSIVE CARE UNIT

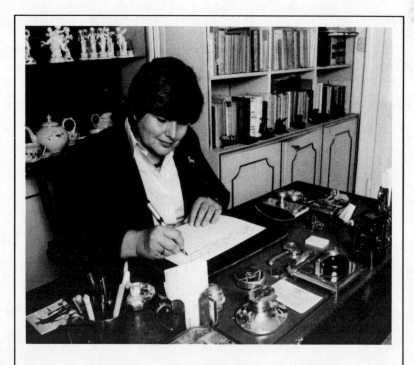

Romana Negri

The Roland Harris Trust Library

THE NEWBORN
IN THE INTENSIVE CARE UNIT
A Neuropsychoanalytic Prevention Model

Romana Negri

Foreword by
Donald Meltzer

edited by
Meg Harris Williams

translated by
Maria Pia Falcone

The Clunie Press

London
KARNAC BOOKS

First published in 1994 by
H. Karnac (Books) Ltd.
58 Gloucester Road
London SW7 4QY

Copyright © 1994 by Romana Negri
Foreword © 1994 by Donald Meltzer
"The Ugly Duckling" © 1994 by Meg Harris Williams

The rights of Romana Negri to be identified as author of this work have .
been asserted in accordance with §§ 77 and 78 of the Copyright
Design and Patents Act 1988.

All rights reserved. No part of this book may be reproduced,
in any form, by any process or technique,
without the prior written permission of the publisher.

British Library Cataloguing in Publication Data

Negri, Romana
   The Newborn in the Intensive Care Unit:
   A Neuropsychoanalytic Prevention Model. —
   (Roland Harris Trust Library)
   I. Title   II. Series
   618.9201

   ISBN: 1 85575 073 2

Printed in Great Britain by BPC Wheatons Ltd, Exeter

In Memory of Martha Harris,
a Master and a friend,
who was able to combine
depth and sharpness of insight in her work
with the gift of her great humanity

FAUST: But I am not searching for salvation through in-
difference; to be greatly moved is the best thing about
being human; and when a man is moved, he senses the
deep and infinite, even though the world makes feeling
difficult for him.

Goethe, *Faust*

ACKNOWLEDGEMENTS

The number of people I wish to thank for helping me with the experience that has gone into this book is very great: firstly, the young patients and their parents; Professor Adriana Guareschi; Federico Bergonzi, the first head physician of the Neonatal Pathology Department; his successor and the current head physician, Luigi Gargantini; and the medical staff: Lina Cazzaniga, Orazio Consolo, Sergio Cornelli, Renato Fenini, Maria Teresa Oggionni, Luigi Re, Franco Suardelli, and Enrica Sampellegrini. I am also greatly indebted to the nursing staff: Giusy Molinai, Piera Zerbi, Danila Pintus, Emanuela Bezza, Antonella Carminati, Rosita Ciocca, Rosanna Facchetti, Vanessa Frau, Angela Garatti, Isabella Guerini Silvia Guarnerio, Graziella Locati, Monica Manetta, Cecilia Marchesi, Anna Maria Martinenghi, Paola Martinenghi, Lucia Mauri, Luciana Metalli, Anna Maria Nardini, Bambina Nesi, Susanna Petrò, Vilma Petrò, Monica Pianazza, Lucia Pizzocchero, Grazia Possenti, Elena Resmini, Cinzia Rota, Elisabetta Simonelli, Serena Tomsic, and Maria Vailati. I also want to express my most sincere thanks to Mrs Dina Vallino for her important contribution in discussing some chapters, and also to Dr Pierandrea Lussana and Mrs Maria Pagliarani Zanetta for this. My heartfelt thanks go to my friends and colleagues, Dr Carla Zilocchi, Dr Adrian Williams, Dr Beppe Campana, Mrs Vilma Colombo, and Dr Simona Nissim, for their patient and thorough work in reading and reviewing the text; and my affectionate gratitude to my sister Pinuccia, to Angelo Gimmillaro my brother-in-law, to Maria and Alba my nieces, for their remarkable hard work in typing and reviewing all the material.

I want to express my particular gratitude to my elder sister Elvira, who died recently. With the generous spirit that characterized her life, she followed my life experiences from the very beginning, in ways useful—indeed, essential—to me. She was a great nature-lover and my first master in the observational field: when we were children she made me know ants and snails in the garden of our house. She then took a degree in natural sciences, and her contribution to my works, and in particular to this one which she saw finished, has been really significant.

Finally, I wish to express my deep gratitude to my parents: to my father, a veterinary surgeon, who taught me, amongst other things, to recognize the importance of observation and of non-verbal communication; and to my mother, a teacher, whom I admire for the respect she has always shown towards the children's world.

CONTENTS

ACKNOWLEDGEMENTS   vii

FOREWORD   xiii
   Donald Meltzer

THE UGLY DUCKLING   xvii
   Meg Harris Williams

Introduction   1

1.   **Work with the parents**   9

     Introduction   9
     The approach with parents   13
     Anxieties about death   16
     The narcissistic wound   18
     The aesthetic conflict   18

The methodology of intervention   20
Interrupted pregnancy   27
The separation–individuation process   30
Catastrophic anxiety and the sense of guilt   35
Conclusions   37
Meeting with parents of children who die   39

2.   **Work with the staff**   **43**

Work method and level   45
Model evolution   45
Theoretical discussion and presentation
of the clinical experience   52

PHASE I
The emotional atmosphere:
the state of paranoid anxiety   53

PHASE II
The concept of the neutral role   59

PHASE III
Mirror resonance:
nurses experience mothers' and children's feelings   71

PHASE IV
Thinking about the work group:
nurses talk about themselves   75
Final conclusions   78

3.   **Infant observation**   **81**

Methodological aspects   82
Difficulties of infant observation in the incubator   84
The first period   88
The child's suffering   90
The child's physiognomy   91

The image of the living child
in the parents' mind   95

The child's states of irritability
and first mental movements:
object differentiation   97

Removal of the tracheal tube:
a second birth   99

The child's abrupt starting;
grasping; the child's sleep   103

The child's first waking moments;
the nurses start to separate from the child   108

The child's first organizational patterns:
32–34 weeks   110

Thought formation:
the integration of sensori-motor experiences
and emotional experiences deriving from
the object relation   113

The mother's depression and its mirror-like
repercussions on the nursing staff;
the emotional experience modulated by the child   118

Splitting:
the toilet breast;
the experience of trusting, of being contained   121

Conclusions   123

4. **The neuropsychological screening
    of the infant
    before its discharge from hospital   131**

    Infant examination   133

5. **Post-discharge follow-up   149**

    Intervention methodology   149

6.   Psychopathological conditions   **157**

Psychopathological risks   157

Early psychoses, or general development disorders,
according to DSM III   165

The psychosomatic syndrome   169

The "minimal brain dysfunction syndrome"   174

7.   Treatment   **183**

Final considerations   194

**8.   The treatment and development
of children with cerebral palsy**   **197**

The child   197

The parents   199

A difficult development   200

Risks involved in the first period   203

The process of separation and individuation   207

The mothers' group   209

The health providers' group   221

REFERENCES AND BIBLIOGRAPHY   223

INDEX   249

FOREWORD

Donald Meltzer

The process of discovery of the borderline between animal and human, between brain and mind, between computation and thought, between facts and meaning, has been a steady one in the field of psychoanalysis. But this relentless progress has separated the movements (not necessarily the institutions) of psychoanalysis and the sciences, including the science of medicine. While the practice of analysis has become more and more self-consciously artistic, medicine has lost its art to the machine and the laboratory. The heart of this divergence lies in the acknowledgement that we are studying events that have at their core essential mystery: that we are only describing and not explaining, for the simple reason that there is nothing to explain. In other words, the field of study of psychoanalysis is a phenomenological one in which elements are bound not by causality, but by pattern and "family resemblances".

When Melanie Klein, as a result of direct observation of children, focussed attention on the first years of life, she not only opened a field of study but also moved the methodology of psychoanalysis back into the realm of the natural sciences, where naming and describing serve the purpose of ordering man's picture of his world. Gradually, over the years, Freud's concern about mental pain and pleasure, as well as his aspiration to cure, have yielded place to concepts about uncertainty, about cognitive development, about the difference between adaptation and emotional development, about confusional states, misconceptions, thought disorder, and the differentiation of "worlds".

In the early days of psychoanalysis it seemed completely reasonable to ask such questions as: "When is the neural apparatus sufficiently developed to enable it to perform certain functions?" This no longer seems a reasonable question, for it has hidden in it a subtext: "When does the tiny animal become a human being?" The wonderful developments in genetic studies have tended to perpetuate both the question and its subtext by allowing the implication that not only bodily structure but also behaviour is programmed by the genes. This elliptical addendum eradicates the mystery of the organism, for it does not admit the non-Darwinian evolution of the forms that generate behaviour. The Darwinian dictum may explain the survival of particular forms, and genetics may provide a mechanism for their reproduction, but they go no distance at all towards exploring the mystery of nature's infinite inventiveness, let alone the aesthetic of living forms.

The babies—the human babies—that Dr Romana Negri has worked with and here describes have indeed been torn into this world half-made-up. But what they lack in physiological equipment can usually be met by the advances of medical science. This book is all about the emotional experience of the baby in this predicament, who has not had enough of one type of life to be able to transfer its emotional allegiances to the new one. The approach to this problem, as it is illustrated here, involves a philosophy that goes far beyond the humane attitude of alleviating suffering which operates in hospital medicine.

Through her work in mother–baby observation under Esther Bick and Martha Harris, supplemented more recently by observational research in foetal behaviour by means of ultrasound, Dr Negri has become deeply engaged in this philosophy of the essential individuality of the human being by virtue of its capacity to have experiences that shape the evolving structure of its person and personality. There is no purpose to be served in asking, "At what point in gestation do experiences—human experiences—begin?" They began many thousands of years ago with the beginnings of symbol formation and the capacity to wonder, to question. Why do not horses speak? It is not part of their natural history—the Wittgensteinian answer. Having experiences is part of the human natural history. Freud struggled a bit with the problem in the "Wolf Man" paper where he found he could not decide at what age the actual observation of the primal scene took place: at 30 months, at 16 months, or at 6 months. What he seems to have realized is that the function we call "memory", as distinct from the computer function of "recall", is an imaginative reconstruction—as Paul Schilder described in *The Image and Appearance of the Human Body*.

One of the amazing and mysterious aspects of mentality is that it makes use of the near-infinite capacity of the human brain for recall. The unconscious availability of recall for imaginative reconstruction as memory is continually being demonstrated in the analytic procedure. The appearance in dreams of items from unconscious observation (the entire sensory field) that have taken on emotional significance in the transference is a continual clinical experience. As Freud pointed out: in the first instance the ego is a body-ego. The neural apparatus records the experiences, but it is the body that has them. The baby "knows" its mother from its nine-months' sojourn in a deeper and more complex sense than it will ever again "know" another being.

The recall of events then serves as the matrix from which the imaginative reconstruction of memories of experiences takes place, thus transferring the venue from brain to mind, from the precision of the computer to the idiosyncratic world(s) of phantasy, available for symbol formation and thought, through dreaming and the creation of meaning. There is no need to ask when this process commences; it is in the tissues that the primary events take place, and in the building of structure—of the body and of the mind—that they are incarnate. Structure *is* memory. Thus it is that man's picture of his world and his story of his personal past is in constant re-construction and modification. Were it not so, psychoanalysis would have no claim to profound modification of the personality. This may seem an excursion into the realm of philosophy of mind, but it is not so. It is a statement of the implications of the development in discovery of the phenomenology of the analytic consulting room, contained in the history of scientist/artists from Freud to Bion.

To return now to the important work of Dr Negri, whose orientation was, as I have said, inspired by her work in mother–baby observation under the tutelage of Esther Bick and Martha Harris, augmented by her experience in recent years of the ultrasonic study of non-identical twins in the womb, followed by mother–baby observation, and continued through the toddler stage into nursery school. These babies were struggling to survive in a new environment for which they were neither physiologically nor emotionally adequately prepared. The central psychological problem to which Dr Negri addressed herself was one that could only be approached from a communal angle: the community of parents, medical staff, nurses. It will be seen that Dr Negri functioned as observer and psychotherapeutic commentator, not as team-leader. She can hardly be said to have initiated anything, but, rather, through her attitude to have encouraged a view of the baby itself as the initiator in its struggle to survive. Even the function of formulation she has left to other participants, so that her own function, above all, is to be seen to respect the baby as initiator.

This attitude has its foundation in a conviction that the life *in utero*, as an experiential world, lies beyond the limits of external-world language. It belongs to the realm of what cannot be said but can only be shown. Wilfred Bion tried to show it in some sections of *The Dawn of Oblivion* (1979) (Volume 3 of his trilogy novel, *A Memoir of the Future*, 1975-81). Meg Harris Williams has done it also in her contribution to this book: borrowing the language of the poets to "show" the mental state of the sojourn traced by Dr Negri for these premature babies.

In summary, what the reader will encounter in this volume, and what Mrs Williams is attempting to show from the baby's point of view, is the struggle to survive with the help of a transitional environment, both physiological and psychological, between life in the womb and life at the breast. It is clearly a no-man's land between the companionship/service of the placenta and the breast/mind of the mother.

The Ugly Duckling

Meg Harris Williams

The morning after the night when I was prematurely ejected from my mother's womb during a violent tempest at the gestational age of 32 weeks and 4 days, I awoke to find myself in many pieces, pinioned to the incubator floor, with my several senses separately trapped in distinct forms of torture: my eyes shut against insufferable brightness, my mouth scorched by dryness, my skin scratched by roughness, the sensitive mucosae of my nose crudely pierced by foreign tubes. Worst of all my ears—the portals of my body's harmony—detected no familiar music, no rhythmic consensus: nothing but a universal blank, with wisdom at all entrances quite shut out. Only pain made any link between my senses so that I could recognize they were all functions of myself, *me*. In contrast to the unnatural alertness of my senses was the moribund heaviness of my body, the deadweight of limbs and extremities which only hours before had danced in the amniotic fluid with surgings of power. Only the night before I had been treading Placenta's comfortable consistence in our waters dark and deep as half on foot, half flying, I explored the universe that had been created for us.

Now, I found myself wrecked on the shore, with every muscle tightly bound and every orifice exposed to the merciless digital probes and arrows of outrageous beings who stabbed relentlessly at my tissues, causing intense pain despite the immature myelinization of my nervous fibres. No longer a swimmer or a flyer, I lay randomly diffused in all directions, unable to prop my languished head. Though in pain, intimate impulse prompted my eyes momentarily to open of their own accord, and despite the terrible blinding light, I glimpsed with awe the huge and wondrous monolithic forms looming over me. My mouth could almost have gasped in amazement, "O brave new world", could indeed have screamed aloud, were it not that my virginal lungs were held in check by an infrasensuous perception of my own: I suddenly divined that according to the colossal all-knowing all-powerful beings who encircled me, I was monstrously ugly, deformed beyond the power of expectation. I was a horrible mistake born of some hideous intercourse, some unnatural conjunction of the stars. The truth was out—I saw it face to face. I was a creature of the dark, taking the horrid form of darkness visible. And because I was a harbinger of death, with death's odour clinging to me, they pierced my nasal passages—an eye for an eye, a tooth for a tooth—and the arrows sunk in deep. I was pinned like Oedipus on Cithaeron. There was no venom in the pain they caused me through the immobilization of my muscles and the burning of my senses, for, clearly, I was not one of their own kind; I did not relish or passion as they. I realized that they were making the preparations for my sacrifice; hence the judgemental severity of those impassive helmeted heads that nodded miles above me.

At this point I believe I must have lapsed into unconsciousness. Certainly it was aeons before I opened my eyes again. That time was spent at first mostly in a state of non-being, when I was perhaps not unconscious but not asleep or awake either, and often exhausted by the meaningless overwhelming stimulation of one or more of my sensuous orifices as fluids were drained in or out of me at feet, nose, or scalp. I was alternately abandoned for timeless periods to wallow in a sensuous desert, and then tossed restlessly on the parching wave of one sense-tip to another, in a way that utterly dislocated my sense of identity. In fact, that was the main cause of my suffering—more than the physical pain (to which I became habituated and which was in any case only intermittent). Yet even when I longed to yield the ghost, the envious air still flooded into my clockwork lungs to insist on my life's mechanical pant; indeed, this now dominated in significance the heartbeat that had always been my personal organic measure of existence. I gave up trying to work out the meaning of all this, or why the preparations for the sacrifice were taking so long—longer than my whole lifetime so far, it seemed. But while fluid still coursed in my veins, however tainted it was by some mysterious leprous distilment of unknown origins, I found myself in calmer moments, through some innate prompting, trying to remember my old life with Placenta in the womb— difficult though it was to use my present experience as a means of recollecting that original world of reality. Perhaps if I could remember what it was like before the shipwreck, I would not be lost in loss itself, condemned to a universe of death where peace and rest could never dwell.

As you can guess from the very fact that I am telling you this story from my now secure and well-established vantage point of three months' post-partum age, being now in complete possession of my mother, I did pull through in the end. Every creature has its home, which gives it its dignity; but after my expulsion I was unhousel'd, disappointing, unanel'd; and my very homelessness showed me to be an ugly, worthless, and insignificant being. Gradually, however, the incubator itself became more like home. My left foot (the one that was not bandaged from heelpricks) began to recognize the smooth hardness of its rounded corner, my buttock to snuggle into the fleecy hollow of the mattress with an almost friendly sensation (though it was a sad change from the buoyancy of my amniotic fluid), and even to enjoy the fluctuations from dryness to wetness and squiggling into it; indeed, I found my muscles now seemed to be mercifully bound with elastic rather than rigid wires. Also there was at times a strange and haunting music, reminding me of a humming that I knew from long ago, but much louder, and which gave delight but hurt not. Another astonishing aid to recollection was an ambrosial wetness that occasionally approached my parched lips and was immediately sucked in greedily by my tongue, just as it had sucked and spouted the amniotic fluid. So I knew there were still riches in heaven. As well as this, I became aware of huge presences brooding motionlessly nearby for long periods, whose mellow omniscient effluence gave me comfort even though I was careful never to open my eyes. These mighty presences seemed to be the source not only of the painful probings to which I was accustomed, but also of other tactile manipulations of a soothing nature, to which I could respond with other pleasant sensations in my tummy and bowels.

It was after a succession of moments like these, which took on the character of a pattern, that a new truth dawned on me: I was not in hell, but in purgatory. For some reason I had been redeemed from death, in spite of my ugliness. My prison sentence was over, and I had entered a chrysalid existence. Now the incubator walls were a permeable membrane that allowed me to ruminate on the scents, sounds, and movements of my life, past and present. These ruminations began during my increasing periods of respite from irritation and dislocation. But it is only now, with mature hindsight, that I can piece together a properly philosophical narrative; and the story of my early life went something as follows.

At the very beginning, then, when the world was created for me shortly after the courtship of my sperm and ovum was consummated, my desire and will were revolved by the love that moves the sun and the other stars; I swam in all directions, and all directions were One. In my boundless wisdom I knew the depth without the tumult of the soul. It seemed I was the first that ever burst into that summer sea. Naturally I was a Pythagorean, guided by my innate sense of harmony, and after each revolution I swam upwards into the sweet-smelling clouds in order to tune my senses to the music of the spheres. It was on one of those regular flights of worshipful exuberance that, to my surprise, I first encountered Placenta, who had been created to be my friend and partner. Very soon I realized how much more satisfactory was mutual exploration than narcissistic reflection; and each day, under the rosy glow that filtered through the eyelids of the womb, we pursued our play hand in hand. How well we came to know and understand the world about us—its contrapuntal rhythms and tastes, pulsations, suckings, and excretions; I measured my newly developing hardnesses against Placenta's responsive soft recesses and convolutions; I timed his reassuring souffle against my own distinct heartbeat, and beyond that, in complex syncopation, the heartbeat and other meaningful rhythms of our eternal Mother. The Sons of Morning sung their solemn music and our fancy was enwrapped. And when the day was over, I floated up into my favourite transverse position, curled over the back of the universe; and Placenta with a weight of pleasure sank down through the clouds and held me like a dream.

You might have thought there was nothing more we could want in life. An infinite variety of sensations were ours, and when the weather was inclement—for even in our womb there were sometimes unpleasant vibrations whose source we could only surmise—we always rode the storm together. If anything, these brief periods of anxiety strengthened our relationship; we were deeply religious and knew everything was conducted in our ultimate interest. We pledged to share our experience in bliss or woe, and I could not imagine our ever being parted. Yet if I recollect clearly, before the great tempest came which shattered our world, there were some rumblings of discontent, some unresolved questionings. For as my own strength and powers increased—as they did steadily—I sensed less willingness on the part of my world to accommodate them: a sort of rebellion, as it were, a jostling for position, even at times a blatant squeezing and constriction that I could no longer interpret as mere playfulness. Somewhere there was hostility. I knew Placenta was not to blame for this, and still every day I journeyed forth, and at eve resumed my position close to him on the back of the universe. But it seemed to me his attitude was becoming more fixed, less imaginative. I wondered if he was capable of the daring strides in speculation that I sometimes found myself engaged in. For by this time I knew our world pretty well, and the pioneering thrill of conquering terra incognita had lost its savour. Rather, I began to feel like the spiritual Cottager who knows that beyond his garden gate there are such things as the Andes and the Burning Mountains with their snowy peaks bright in the sunlight. On top of this, I had qualms about outside elements coming in, wafted on some dubious wave, encroaching on our narrow limits. I began to have suspicions about a third party impinging on our room, in mutual amity too straight, too close. Or possibly more than one: my fertile imagination suggested—and I shuddered to conceive of it—that the seas might be thronged with spawn innumerable.

Were any of these warning signs? I still don't know the answer, or if it would have made any difference. For it is certain that nothing in my tentative fond surmises prepared me for the sudden tempest in which Placenta and I were separated and lost, sent with hideous ruin and combustion down to bottomless perdition. In the terrible confusion of that roar and rout I don't know which of us was expelled first, but my head was rammed into the abyss, and as the life fluids were crushed out of me I saw Placenta in my mind's eye, his visage shattered by forced fingers rude and sent down the stream in bloody spongiform strips. Grim were the punishments meted out to those as evidently ugly and sinful as I knew I must be, left stranded on the shore to be swept by parching winds; while Placenta, I was sure, was discarded to become an island salt and bare, a mere quintessence of dust.

During the following aeons, I suffered in the ways that I have already attempted to describe to you. There was one additional factor in my distress, which even now, secure in my rightful empire, I am not sure I have fully catharsized: was there any truth in my speculation that if not Placenta, then some other One, ousted me from my first home? Was that other One perhaps of nobler birth than me (a mere creature of earth), the one They really wanted, even though my ugliness was later redeemed and forgiven? The question arises, indeed, as to who occupies my first home now? Happiest are those who seek to know no more. Suffice it here to swiftly bring my history— which, as you know, is a happy one—to a close, on an optimal note.

For despite the traumatic conclusion of my tale-within-a-tale, this recollection of my early life seemed to have a healing effect on my critical condition as I lay in the incubator. The process of anamnesis reminded me that my severed senses once had their origin in an organic reality that was me, myself, and that my feeble muscular movements were also, however poor, mine own. Then, strange as it was, the priestly manipulations of the shadowy godlike beings stationed near me increasingly had the effect not of squashing me but of motivating my powers to function independently, even to express distinct propositions. The experience again became mine of more than one sense acting in unison, or at least relatedly, such as when my tongue sucked and my deepest bowels rumbled affectionately in response. To my joy I came to realize that, leading with my left foot, I could swivel my entire body round, until I was lying crosswise from side to side in the incubator, touching at head and feet, just as I had used to lie across the top of the uterus. Placenta had gone for ever, sunk beneath the watery floor; but my horizons had opened, and I began to believe that perhaps another friend might be found.

At the gestational age of 36 weeks and 2 days I reached the turning-point. Even before they came to extubate me, I was conscious of a strange thrill of anticipation, of rousing motions within me which disposed my preconceptions to something extraordinary. I felt barely a pinprick as the familiar tube was withdrawn, and there was only time for a split-second of panic and remorse as I realized how attached I had become to it, when with a sharp intake of breath my lungs filled my chest and head with the delicious taste of empyreal air—tempered by the immortals and never known by me till now. Clouds of glory issued from my whole being: my joy was so intense, bursting its grape against my palate fine, that I knew death could not be far away. Still I demanded one more favour from the archangelic Muse that supported me in the large recompense of its hands. As the hands stroked a line down my back from the nape of my neck, I was struck by the inspiration that I was a creature with a spine, an endoskeleton, an internally sustained identity; and all my senses at once sprang into order at the angelic command. To my terror I realized my eyes were about to open yet once more. I knew it must be death to presume to look into the heaven of heavens. But I had to know. I opened my eyes; I saw the bright stars that flamed in the forehead of the morning sky. In the midst of the dazzling white radiance that enveloped me closely, my mouth latched on to the nipple which was at its core. Simultaneously, the angel looked homeward into my heart of hearts, and I saw that I was a beautiful baby.

Quotes in order of appearance

Shakespeare, *The Tempest*; Milton, "insufferably bright"; Milton, *Lycidas*, "trembling ears", 77; Milton, *Paradise Lost*, "wisdom at one entrance quite shut out", "universal blank of nature's works", III.50; *Paradise Lost*, "Treading the crude consistence, half on foot, half flying", II.941; *Paradise Lost*, "man he made, and for him built/Magnificent this world", IX.152; Swift, *Gulliver's Travels*; Shakespeare, *Hamlet*, "slings and arrows of outrageous fortune", III.i.58; Milton, *Samson Agonistes*, "he lies at random, carelessly diffused,/With languished head unpropped", 118–119; *Paradise Lost*, "though in pain", I.125; *Samson Agonistes*, "intimate impulse", 223; *The Tempest*, "brave new world", V.i.183; Shakespeare, *King Lear*, Edmund's speech, I.ii.1–22, and "whoremaster man to lay his goatish disposition to the charge of a star"; Bible, St Paul to Corinthians: "in a glass darkly . . . face to face"; *Paradise Lost*, "darkness visible", I.63, "horrid", "burning marle"; *Lycidas*, "welter to the parching wind", "whelming tide", "where'er thy bones are hurled", 13, 155; Shakespeare, *Richard III*, "yield the ghost, but still the envious flood/Stopped in my soul", I.iv.36; *Hamlet*, "leprous distilment . . . courses through/The natural gates and alleys of the body", I.v.63–67; Plato, *Phaedrus*, "every soul has by nature beheld true being . . . but not every soul finds it easy to use its present experience as a means of recollecting the world of reality."; *Paradise Lost*, "lost in loss itself . . . universe of death where peace and rest can never dwell", I.66, 525; Keats, *Fall of Hyperion*, "every creature hath its home", I.171; *Hamlet*, "unhousel'd, disappointed, unanel'd", I.v.77; *The Tempest*, "sounds and sweet airs that give delight and hurt not . . . hum about mine ears", "riches ready to drop upon me", III.ii.133–140; *Paradise Lost*, "Dove-like satst brooding on the dark abyss", I.21, "effluence of essence increate", III.6; *Fall of Hyperion*, "and still these two were postured motionless", I.85; Keats, "Ode to Autumn", "sitting careless on a granary floor . . . watches the last oozings hours by hours"; Wordsworth, *The Prelude*, "huge and mighty forms", I.425, "ye presences of nature", I.490, II; Dante: hell, purgatory, heaven; Keats, *Letters*, letter to Reynolds, 11 July 1819, "chrysalis with two loopholes for eyes"; Dante, end of *Paradiso*, "my desire and will were revolved by the love that moves the sun and the other stars"; Bion, *Memoir of the Future, Book III*, "courtship of sperm and ovum"; Wordsworth, *Laodamia*, "depth and not the tumult of the soul"; Coleridge, *Ancient Mariner*, "the first that ever burst into that silent sea"; Milton, "On the Harmony of the Spheres"; Meltzer, *The Apprehension of Beauty*, Placenta's "reassuring souffle", "ugly clown", p. 43; *Paradise Lost*, IV, creation of Eve, "hand in hand", 321, harmony of day and night; *Lycidas*, "under the opening eyelids of the morn", 26; Milton, "At a Solemn Musick" and the "Nativity Ode", "fancy was enwrapped"; *Phaedrus*, souls on the back of the universe; Wordsworth, *Prelude*, "weight of pleasure . . . held me like a dream", II.177–180; Shakespeare, *Antony and Cleopatra*, "infinite variety", II.ii.236; *Paradise Lost*, "share in bliss or woe", IX.831; Bronte, *Wuthering Heights*, separation of Cathy and Heathcliff; Keats, *Letters*, letter to Rice, 24 March 1818, "spiritual cottager . . ."; *Paradise Lost*, "dubious wave", "narrow limits", "our room", "mutual amity . . . too strait, too close", II.1042, IV.360; Milton, *Comus*, "thronging the seas with spawn innumerable", 713; *Paradise Lost*, "bottomless perdition" I.45, "roar and rout" (also *Lycidas*); *Lycidas*, "forced fingers rude . . . down the stream", 4, 62; *Paradise Lost*, Eden an "island salt and bare", XI.830; *Paradise Lost*, "creature formed of earth", IX.149, "instead of us outcast . . . mankind created", IV.106; *King Lear*, Edmund and Gloucester—"smell a fault . . . ", I.i.16; *Paradise Lost*, IV.774, "happiest if ye seek to know no more"; Plato, the *Phaedrus*, anamnesis (remembering reality); Shakespeare, *As You Like It*, "poor but mine own", V.iv.57; Keats, Notes on Milton, on Milton's "stationing"; *Lycidas*, "sunk beneath the watery floor", 167; *Paradise Lost*, "into the heaven of heavens I have presumed, and drawn empyreal air, thy tempering", VII.12; Wordsworth, *Immortality Ode*, "trailing clouds of glory"; *Samson Agonistes*, "rousing motions . . . dispose/To something extraordinary my thoughts", 1382–1383; Keats, "Ode on Melancholy", "burst joy's grape . . ."; *Lycidas*, "in thy large recompense be good/To all that wander in that perilous flood", 184–185; Keats, "Ode to Apollo", "that terrific band—spring forward", "powers of song combine"; *Lycidas*, "yet once more"; "sun flames in the forehead of the morning sky", "look homeward angel", 1,171,163; *Hamlet*, Hamlet to Horatio: "passion's slave . . . heart of hearts", III.ii.71–73.

THE NEWBORN
IN THE INTENSIVE CARE UNIT

INTRODUCTION

The present work originated in an experience with the Neonatal Pathology Division of the Hospital of Treviglio–Caravaggio (Bergamo), where I have now been working for 18 years as an Infant Neuropsychiatric Consultant on the basis of an agreement between the Local Health Unit No. 32 and the University of Milan.

The request for the intervention of an infant neuropsychiatrist, which was initially aimed at the early detection of cerebral palsy, was made in December 1976; but already in 1977, as a consequence of follow-up checks after discharge, the case analysis of young patients hospitalized during 1977 (Negri, 1980) showed a significant incidence of features, phobias, and other fears recognizable as typical warning symptoms of a psychopathological nature (Table 1).

The phobias of being undressed and of "having one's feet, hands, or head touched, and the 'little hat' phobias", are, I believe, particularly related to emotional experiences derived from therapies involving drips into the scalp and frequent heel-pricks for the taking of blood, and in general to the traumas

1

TABLE 1
Alarm symptoms

- averting the gaze
- pretending to sleep
- looking secretly when you're not being looked at
- absence of smiling
- stiff mimicry
- sound and movement stereotypes (such as repetitive hand gestures, etc.)
- excessive or strange interest in movements of the tongue in the mouth
- tremor (especially during the first two months)
- hiccuping (especially during the first two months)
- motor restlessness
- postural anomalies
- psychosomatic manifestations at cutaneous or respiratory level
- phobia of having the feet or hands touched
- "little-hat" phobia (fear of having the head stroked)
- fear of being undressed
- other fears
- feeding disorders
- major alterations in biological rhythms (most frequent manifestations: sleep disorders; irritability)

---

and manipulations to which these young patients are subjected (Earnshaw, 1981; Lezine, 1977, Szure, 1981).

These findings are understandable if we take into account the significance of mental life not only at birth but also during pregnancy, as confirmed by neurophysiological, psychoanalytic, and ultrasonic studies. Great importance is attached to the way in which the baby lives the first period of its life, which then reflects on its future development. Moreover, in the fields of neonatology and anaesthesia, several studies have been carried out on the suffering experienced by the child in relation to its pathology and to the invasive therapeutic procedures. These are recent findings (Gasparoni et al., 1990; McGrath, 1987; Orzalesi, Maffei, De Caro, Pellegrini-Caliumi, 1989; Porter, 1989; Sumner, 1993); until a few years ago (and this was reassuring for the nursing staff) it was assumed that the paucity of cutaneous nociceptive sense receptors in the newborn, the poor myelinization of nervous fibres, and subcortical reflex-responses implied a low perception of the painful stimulus. Therefore, the behaviour of the child was not seriously considered as a means of communication. Crying, for instance, was regarded as a reflex (aspect of neurological semiology).

Saint-Anne Dargassies (1974) defines a peculiar kind of crying of the newborn, which is "irritating to hear", as a symptom of severe cerebral suffering. This important neurologist thus gives an interesting description of the peculiarly intense suffering experienced by the pathological newborn: this kind of crying is so charged with anxiety that it is difficult for the adult (who finds it "irritating to hear") to tolerate and understand it.

Research emphasizes that the newborn's existential condition during its early life is closely linked to the manner of interaction between it and its mother, and also that the first interactive processes play a significant role in the infant's future development. I would like to refer to a few authors:

Kennell, Trause, and Klaus (1975) stress the existence of maternal emotive–affective sensitization soon after delivery. Klaus and Kennell (1983a, 1983b) describe orderly sequences, which are strong emotional vehicles in the mother's behaviour immediately after birth. Schaffer (1974), Brazelton et al. (1975), and Papousek and Papousek (1979) refer to the mutual interaction of mother and newborn with its self-adjusting characteristics. Leiderman et al. (1973) and Leiderman and Seashore (1974) point out the alteration of this function consequent on a separation of mother and child during the early days. Dunn (1980) stresses the newborn's ability to stimulate affective responses by the mother through its earliest feeding behaviour. Similarly, Thomas (1963) points out that these derive also from the newborn's ability to communicate its needs and condition.

Furthermore, according to Brody (1956), the mother's presence stimulates the newborn's visual attention, and handling activates the newborn's special sense endings (tactile receptors). Moreover, Brazelton et al. (1975) stress that the sensory input in the newborn is organized in terms of time through the harmonious cyclic modulation and integration of waking states. As far as the sensory aspect is concerned, already during the neonatal period—but also during life *in utero*—the olfactory discriminatory skills are already developed, thus allowing the newborn to single out the mother's breast smell (McFarlane, 1975), as are also the gustatory discriminatory skills, thus allowing it to distinguish the taste of milk as well as of other liquids (Johnson & Salisbury, 1975).

It is clear that the newborn admitted to the intensive care unit is exposed to a serious threat regarding its chance of acquiring the attributes studied by the above-mentioned researchers. It therefore became necessary to start a thorough and more detailed process of prevention. I have defined the measures I adopted as direct and indirect "preventive environmental actions" (Table 2).

It must not be forgotten that when these preventive actions were implemented, they were intended for newborn infants who in one way were subjected to hyperstimulation (Gottfried & Gaiter, 1985), but in another way suffered from serious deficiencies (Berrini & Carati, 1977). This is why it was stressed that it was a priority for parents to come close to the child from the very beginning of its hospitalization. At the same time, the need emerged to arrange meetings with the medical and nursing staff working within the Unit. The work carried out with parents and with the medical and nursing staff over these years has allowed me to widen the scope and change the nature of the preventive actions according to the specific situation of the individual newborn (Negri, 1992).

It is difficult to identify systematically how much of the therapeutic effect is attributable to nurses and how much to parents. A close integration between the contributions of both was established, as well as a sort of "mutual feeding" aimed at best meeting the infant's needs. Nevertheless, in order to provide a more systematic presentation, the therapeutic actions will be described separately.

TABLE 2
Preventive environmental actions

I. Indirect actions

   a. *on parents*

      interviews from the first days of the child's hospitalization, near the incubator; and interviews away from the child

   b. *on medical and non-medical staff*

      i. free-subject weekly group meetings

      ii. filling in and discussing an ad hoc form

      iii. discussion of observation material

      iv. "open-door" observation of the preterm newborn

      v. participation in the children's follow-up after discharge

II. Direct actions on the child in the incubator

   a. *observation*

   b. *posture*

   c. *light adjustment device to reduce light intensity*

   d. *dressing the baby from early on in coloured wool hat and socks*

   e. *cutaneous stimulation:* lambskin undersheet; gentle and slow massage by parents or nurses; positioning mothers' or nurses' hands during feeding in a "containing" way

   f. *acoustic stimulation:* verbal messages from parents or nurses through the incubator opening; sound therapy (introducing into the incubator a recording of the maternal heart beat as received by the baby *in utero*; or of a tape recorded by parents)

   g. *taste stimulation:* by means of a piece of gauze soaked in sweetened water; rose hip syrup on the nurse's or mother's little finger or on the teat of a very small dummy belonging to a *"Nata ora"* ("newborn") doll

TABLE 2
Preventive environmental actions (*continued*)

h. *non-nutritional sucking*

i. proprioceptive and vestibular stimulations: hammock

j. *vestibular stimulation:* oscillations from head to feet
produced by rhythmical pressure on the water
mattress on which the baby lies

k. weaning from the respirator helped by respiratory
re-education: "stretching" the thorax; "body scheme"

III. Actions on the child in the lower-dependency room

a. particular attention paid by the nursing staff to
emotional problems during their routine care of the
child

b. food given by the mother or father; parents are also
invited to visit their child between meals

c. skin-to-skin contact between parents and child: the
naked child is given "kangaroo care"—positioned
against the mother's or father's chest, wrapped around
by a blanket

d. supplementary breast-feeding: enabling the mother to
feed her preterm newborn at the breast even when she
has insufficient milk; also for children having sucking
difficulties; training to suck from the breast

e. developing a "rehabilitation attitude" in mothers and
nurses towards children who are seriously affected
neurologically, under the supervision of a
physiotherapist

IV. Actions on the child after discharge
follow-up

The preventive actions, which are specifically intended for the newborn, are based on infant observation, including all those measures aimed at helping the newborn find hospitalization more tolerable. The most meaningful ones, during the initial period, are such things as: a more satisfactory posture, a means of adjusting the ambient light, a lamb's fleece, fondling, "sound" therapy, taste stimulation, non-nutritional sucking, a water mattress, etc. (see Martin, Herrell, & Rubin, 1979; Scott, Cole, Lucas, & Richards, 1983; Scott & Martin, 1981; Burns, Deddish, Burns, & Hatcher, 1983; De Casper & Fifer, 1980; Field et al., 1986; White & Labarba, 1976; Field et al., 1982; Korner, 1986).

It is clear that deciding on the timing of the above actions is a sensitive problem. Every child, even a newborn, is different from any other child; and in this particular field the child's gestation age and clinical condition makes timing even more crucial and precludes easy schematizations (Als, 1986). We discovered that the way to find the most suitable programme of preventive environmental action was through *infant observation*.

Work with the parents

Introduction

The post-partum days of a pregnancy are critical for the mother psychologically as well as physiologically: in reviewing the experience of giving birth, from the original phantasies of conception and pregnancy to the relationship with the newborn infant. During this stage the feelings and expectations that once focused on the future baby become blurred owing to the emergence of infantile parts of the self; these ask to be contained and comforted, in order that the woman's natural maternal instinct can express itself in her relationship with the baby. The baby needs to be fed, supported, and comforted by its mother in order to begin its new existence. This is a very critical time for the woman, who is in a fragile condition: "that very special condition which is similar to an illness even though it's perfectly normal", as Winnicott (1958) writes. This state should gradually disappear after a few days or weeks, thanks also to the relationship that is established between the mother and the newborn ("breast relationship" and "holding") and to their mutual adjustment.

During pregnancy an internal rethinking process (at instinctual and phantasy level) takes place, moving from an initial narcissistic–fusional position to object investment with the progressive flowing of the woman's interest from herself to the child, which is perceived as being different from herself. Narcissism and the initial mechanisms of idealization and projective identification (the product of conception being confused with parts of the woman's body and with the expectations of the narcissistic self) gradually become less intense, with the progressive joining of mature and infantile parts of the self (maternal self and infantile self) in the woman, then with the acceptance of the child's separateness, which occurs with the physical caesura of childbirth, and eventually with the establishment of the new relationship with the newborn baby.

This is a process that can release ancient conflicts with the internal objects, and all the anxieties and disappointment resulting from the loss of fusion and omnipotence, as well as the anxieties and suffering of separation and depression. The process is accomplished, however, through the joining together of the woman's infantile and maternal parts of the self, leading to the emergence of the maternal availability that gives the woman her natural orientation towards her child. And during this process, from the beginning of pregnancy until the child's first weeks of life, the woman must relive and abandon a part of her own infantile experience and expectations ("abandon memory and desire", as Bion, 1967b, would say), in order to become caring and to love her child in its present reality. Gradually the mutual emotional experience of the breast relationship will lead to an identification with the child that is more mature and serene than that during the period immediately following the birth. It will also lead to the acceptance of a future and of needs that do not necessarily coincide with the phantasies and illusions of pregnancy.

In the framework of mutual adjustment and satisfaction, trying to meet the needs of the newborn, the woman acquires the identity of a "good-enough" mother, identified with and supported by a "good internal mother", which would also find support in the existence of a good external reality during the puerperium period and in the maternity ward itself (see Berrini

& Carati, 1982; Elkan, 1981; Kennell et al., 1991; Klaus, Kennell, Robertson, & Sosa, 1980; Sosa et al., 1980).

Yet if the child is separated from the mother soon after childbirth (as may happen for various reasons), even for a short time, a significant interference with the above process takes place, with potentially depressive implications for the couple. And the child's hospitalization in the intensive care unit, especially when it is seriously preterm or affected by a severe disorder, produces an intense emotional upset, which involves not only the mother–child couple but the father as well. This event is a real trauma for the parents and causes an abrupt disruption of the family plans, which may not be the same for both parents but will have different characteristics according to their specific situations—the mother's in particular.

Sometimes the birth of a seriously preterm child can be the first experience of parenthood for a young couple. When a couple are very close and in agreement about starting a family, the child is "the person" who provides parents with the opportunity to "become a family", to carry on developing, and to have "another life opportunity" (Brazelton, 1981). When conceiving a child, they wish it to be the expression of their own and of their parents' best qualities. Furthermore, the child is seen as the means of achieving a more complete harmony.

Similar feelings may motivate close couples to have further children. Yet the child in need of being hospitalized in a neonatal intensive care unit is not always part of a family project. In socially less favoured couples or especially in couples affected by drug addiction problems, pregnancy and the birth of a child generally can be just physical acts that are not preceded by a thinking process. In such cases, the birth of a preterm child can be the event that for the first time dramatically confronts the parents with the existence of and responsibility for a child, and they find it frightening and oppressing.

Indeed, as far as a large number of preterm newborns are concerned, no rich and hopeful family project is visible, and mothers have often previously undergone several miscarriages or delivered other preterm infants who have eventually died during the neonatal period. In such situations, the child's birth is generally preceded by intense anxiety, and the desire for a new pregnancy is rarely the result of working through the mourning for the previously miscarried newborns. The new child is usually desired more as a replacement of the previous one, as an attempt to deny the interrupted pregnancy (Reid, 1993).

The mother of Alberico, a 7-month preterm infant, expressed herself as follows after five previous miscarriages:

"After all the miscarriages, I felt I was a failure, unable to have children. Even with this child, I was always afraid of losing him, and then I suffered for not carrying him to term. I don't know why, I have always wanted another pregnancy—maybe it was the wish to have something I couldn't have.

I've never analysed why I was doing it, why I persisted with all those examinations—even before I had Alberico, who then arrived by chance, even though I had done nothing to avoid it. It must surely have been an unsatisfied desire for maternity. After a miscarriage, I started all over again; I went on and always suffered. I was upset if I saw a pregnant woman. I had a miscarriage in September. In February my sister-in-law became pregnant; I cried. Even when I became pregnant with Alberico and my stomach grew, I was not happy, I was not convinced; it was probably the fear of losing him. It's strange, because even then, whenever I saw pregnant women I envied them. At the seventh month, I no longer feared losing him, but I was not serene, even though I could feel him; I was always tense, and I said to myself—I don't feel him enough, or too much.

I should have met you before, doctor. I tried, though, to be calm. I could have enjoyed my pregnancy much more. I went to bed early, I rested, but I felt tired, maybe because I was already forty."

So even though the family framework within which the seriously preterm or the high-risk newborn is conceived varies from case to case, there are some emotional features that are the same for all these parents and which become more or less dramatic according to their personality structure.

The approach with parents

It should be stated in advance that, thanks to the cultural roots of this work—which may be traced back to the early 1950s (Prugh, 1953) and to the head physician's special sensitivity— mothers at the Treviglio–Caravaggio Hospital had been allowed since 1972 to come into direct contact with their child. This was initially for breast-feeding mothers and was later extended to all mothers, but was in any case limited to the period of time that the infant was spending in the lower-dependency room of the unit.

From 1978 on I invited parents to stay close to their child for as long as possible during the day from the beginning of hospitalization. In fact, the parents' early closeness to their child is significant not only for the nature of the attachment, with which much literature has been concerned (see Bowlby, 1958; Brazelton, 1981; Ive-Kropf, Negroni, & Nordio, 1976; Klaus & Kennell, 1983a; Robson & Moss, 1970), but also, it seems, to avoid the development of tainted perceptions of the baby. The phantasies evoked by premature birth are increased by the menacing and unfamiliar presence of the department's technical equipment and by common superstitions regarding the future development of a premature baby (Lombardi & Argese, 1982).

Broussard and Martner (1970) confirmed the relationship existing between early maternal perceptions and subsequent child development by remarking on the higher incidence of emotional disorders in children born at term and examined at the age of 4½, whose mothers—a month after delivery— had judged their child to be altogether inferior to the average baby. Yet such a feeling is readily found in parents—especially mothers—of babies in intensive care units, who generally have to face a deeply depressive situation. Observing the attitudes, feelings, and behaviour of the parents of high-risk newborns, Benfield, Leib, and Reuter (1976) found clear reactions of pain and anxiety in the majority of cases—particularly in mothers—

that were similar to those of parents whose children had not survived. According to these authors there is a sense of anticipatory anxiety present, particularly after birth and immediately before leaving the hospital. The intensity of anxiety is not directly proportional to the seriousness of the newborn's illness, but relates to its need of either a respiratory treatment or of some traumatizing treatment.

The observations made by Klaus and Kennell (1970) are also very interesting: they compare the behaviour of mothers who had babies born at term with other mothers who had premature babies. These authors noticed that the first group of mothers behaved in an orderly and foreseeable way with their child in terms of "limb contact", "body caressing", and "glance seeking". But the mothers of premature babies showed a retarded evolution and an erratic mode of contact. The authors found an explanation for this in the precarious health of premature babies who seem almost unable to survive, in the late contact made with the mother, and in the lack of experience owing to the barrier represented by the incubator.

It is not accidental that the "battered baby" syndrome involves twice as many babies who had experienced a long period in hospital, separated from their mothers or parents (Klein & Stern, 1971). In these cases, emotional difficulties emerge in the form of an attitude towards the child, as a result of a defective evolution in the "maternal attachment process" as it has been studied by Bowlby (1958) in the United Kingdom, by Klaus and Kennell (1983b) and Robson (1967) in the United States, and by Ive-Kropf et al. (1976) in Italy.

The parents' early closeness to their child is significant not only for the parents' emotional state but also for the child's physical and mental condition. In this context, Minde (Minde et al., 1980) has pointed out that the newborns who kept their eyes open were most often those who had been most handled and cuddled by their mothers. (This finding is not fully confirmed by my personal experience—see Box 8, page 94. In fact, there are children who, though closely followed by their parents with love and care, spend most of their time sleeping, especially during the first stages of their hospitalization—a sort of "protective apathy", as Tronick, Scanlon, & Scanlon, 1990, define it.) The same author (Minde et al., 1988) has also found a correlation between the child's motor activity and maternal smiles and handling. Moreover, Klaus and Kennell (1983b) underline that, generally speaking, premature newborns who are handled, lulled, fondled, or caressed frequently during their hospitalization exhibit considerably fewer apnoea attacks, and have better weight growth, a lower number of evacuations, and a higher development of certain functions of the nervous system, which persist for a short period even after discharge and return home. Fau (1973) suggests the existence of a relation between feeding in the incubator without any contact and the rise of early and massive anorexia associated with the mother's need and desire to recover the time lost.

Starting in September 1982, I organized a series of interviews during the days immediately following childbirth, first with mothers and later with both parents of the newborn patients, aimed at helping them to work out their anxiety and also at establishing their relationship with the child (Marazzini & Mazzucchelli, 1990; Satge & Soulé, 1976). Bearing in mind the importance of the role played by the staff with respect to the child's health, the importance of the psychological state of the parents, and the importance of the conflict that often characterizes the staff and parents' emotional relationship, I decided to involve the medical staff of the whole department in this new work (Paludetto, 1977). During our weekly meetings, therefore, we discussed the material of the parents' interviews in order to try to understand the defensive mechanisms they might be using—such as denial or splitting and projection (this last often being acted out in relation to the medical and non-medical staff taking care of the child). In this way the staff were placed in a position to understand better the situation they were involved in, rather than having to act out through it.

In addition to this, discussion and comment on the observation sessions led to the increase and improvement of preventive actions. At the suggestion of one nurse, I thought of offering the interview not only to the mothers but also to the fathers, who are invited to the meeting together. The following is a part of a session concerning Pino, a little boy born at 33 weeks, which was the object of discussion in the nurses' group, and after this observation the need emerged to invite fathers to the meetings along with their wifes.

> The mother and father arrive at the consultation. I introduce myself. The father teasingly says that this child will not grow, and he repeats this often, addressing himself to me also. The mother, however, answers that it is not true, that he has gained 100 g over the past few days. Then she puts her hands in the cot, lifts the baby, and sits him down. The father just taps at the incubator glass, trying to call the little boy's attention; then, looking at him, he says that "his face is not formed yet".
> (Observer: G. Odone)

A psychoanalytic approach was used in these interviews, lasting about one hour and giving free play to the parents' communications, so that they could express their experiences and their phantasies. In particular those parents whose children were admitted to hospital for only minor disorders communicated not only anxiety but also phantasies linked to more essential features of pregnancy. One mother reported that her elder child had asked her if the little brother, who was still in her tummy, had a little knife to use to get himself out of it and see the light of day.

Yet reflecting carefully on this type of work made me understand that offering this type of intervention indiscriminately to all parents of newborn patients could be dangerous: some of them, in fact, might experience it as evidence that their child's illness was extremely serious, even if admission was only owing to some minor disease. For this reason, during a routine weekly meeting with the staff of the department, it was decided to offer interviews only to those parents of severely preterm newborns who manifest particularly deep depressive states.

Anxieties about death

Even when carefully adjusted to the various individual situations, however, this intervention did not appear to answer sufficiently to the proposed aim. In fact, it did not help these anxiety-swept parents to distinguish adequately how much of their anxiety was owing to their personal experience and how much to their feeling that the child was in danger of death.

The birth of a seriously preterm or a high-risk infant stirs death anxieties in the parental couple, rooted in the fear of imminent death of their parental as well as of their childish part—neither of which is initially distinguished from the newborn in danger. During this first period, parents report dreams in which much blood is in evidence. One preterm newborn's mother reported that after the first threatened abortion during her pregnancy, she had started "always dreaming of blood, I saw blood everywhere". After the child was born, dreams no longer concerned herself, but the child: "I always saw it regurgitate blood." Indeed, if she saw anything on her baby that could be related to blood, she would be upset all day long. Another preterm child's father reported nightmares with a great deal of blood; one night he dreamt that he was cutting some meat and there was a lot of blood; he suddenly woke up sitting on the bed. In a subsequent stage, the anxiety from experiencing the child as in danger of death can be so extreme that it helps one to understand the parents' trouble in coming near their child, and why they often prefer to stay away from the incubator.

Here is how the mother of Maria, a girl born by Caesarean section at 30 weeks, weighing 800 g, illustrates the problem:

"Then, after she was born, I didn't see her; the next day I went up to see her in a wheel-chair, carrying my intravenous drip—because when they do the Caesarean, they give you a drip for three days—and I saw her very small, ugly; I had a very unpleasant and painful feeling. Fortunately I had my husband near me, who was already attached to the girl; because I was worried and disappointed. I am sure we had a beautiful relationship before; but I must say I thought my husband was fabulous. Besides being very important for me, I believe he is also going to be very important for the girl. It was he who made me notice how beautiful Maria was, even from behind the glass."

One can see clearly here how the death anxieties—the "ugly" death projected into the child—come to the parents by means of "the unpleasant and painful feeling of seeing the child very small and very ugly and feeling worried and disappointed about this".

The narcissistic wound

At this point a more general problem arises, concerning the meaning of what is usually called the "narcissistic wound", which defines what the parents feel when they give birth to a handicapped child (Lax, 1972). Is this, then, a wound inflicted on the narcissism of a couple who have not created a very beautiful creature corresponding to their baby ideal; or is it an experience that is essentially connected with the projection of the "ugly death" into the baby, who is being seen as ugly?

The aesthetic conflict

It is well known from the literature that the emaciated appearance of the premature infant entails important repercussions on the parents' emotional situation, which often weighs very unfavourably on the child's development.

Meltzer (Meltzer & Harris Williams, 1988) has clarified and deepened our view of this problem through his theory of the "aesthetic conflict". According to him, in the very early stages of development it is important to consider the visual aesthetic impact perceived by the baby when it first emerges from the womb and makes contact with the world: "At the beginning was the aesthetic object and the aesthetic object was the breast and the breast was the world." The aesthetic impact experienced in connection with the mother, with her external beauty centred in her breast and in her face, complicated by nipples and eyes, bombards the baby with an emotional experience that is passionate in its nature. In the same way the mother seems to be ravished by the beauty of her baby, and they both become lost in the reciprocal aesthetic impact.

This experience, which is very important for the child's mental evolution, then encounters conflict owing to the fact that it is able to see the goodness and beauty of the object in its exterior qualities, but is unable to know what is hiding inside it. The desire to know the inside—when aimed at discovering the good things—would constitute the basis of an interest in scientific research; whereas curiosity of a mainly intrusive character would produce an interest that is more oriented towards technology. The aesthetic experience that is not accompanied by a desire to penetrate the object would be the basis for development of the child's artistic qualities. "The impact of interferences such as prematurity, permanence in the incubator, early separation, difficulty in breast-feeding, baby's or mother's physical illness" therefore shows up in character development as clearly as tree-ring faults point to past periods of drought.

According to Meltzer, autistic children are not so much disturbed by the absence as by the presence of their maternal object, whose beauty is simultaneously ravishing and perturbing, yet not sufficiently responsive and attentive for them. They are concerned about the interior of the object, which appears so inscrutable owing to the contrast between its external beauty and its expected internal benevolence.

It is necessary to fight for the recognition that the period of maximum beatification between mother and child takes place very early and is soon clouded by various degrees of post-partum depression in the mother and by the child's reaction against the "aesthetic impact" (Meltzer & Harris Williams, 1988). In line with Bion's ideas, Meltzer underlines the pregnancy of the emotional component of this experience, which implies the existence in the child of "a passion for life, a passion for human relations" (Meltzer & Harris Williams, 1988).

I believe that the problem of beauty is a vitally relevant consideration within the sphere of intervention with these very young children. Here one can see clearly how a child's "beauty and weight" are directly related to its viability.

The methodology of intervention

The words of Maria's mother, therefore, express the priority of her need to be helped to look at her very small girl not with the eye that sees death, but with the eye that—through a paternal intervention such as the one her husband was able to offer her—will encourage her to establish a "unique, intimate, direct" link with her child, through the possibility of recognizing in it the features of a pretty and vital girl. But this is not enough. Maria's mother adds again: "Here it is, then; I also wanted to ask you how one can get in touch with a girl even in such difficult conditions, when amongst other things, anxiety is also increased by the presence of so many machines that just scare you. . . ."

These words help us to understand how important it is that mothers or both parents be allowed to live near their child for a large part of the day. Helped by the department's staff, parents must be placed in a position where they do not feel passive or tolerated but, rather, cooperate in the assistance plan organized for their child. This means making them responsible in certain limited fields, such as allowing them to check the correct functioning of the equipment, the regular flow of infusional treatments and continuous feeding, and noting the child's possible responses. (To confirm what has been stated, I would like to quote the experience of the mother of a little girl born at 30 weeks, weighing 1.300 kg. During the follow-up visits, the woman told me that during the baby's hospitalization in the neonatal intensive care unit, her husband had had nightmares, because he could do nothing to help her, unlike his wife, who gave the baby milk. He used to dream that "blood came out of his little daughter's nails, as though it was spilling out". This was a distressing recurrent dream, which ended after he had had the opportunity to give blood to his daughter through a transfusion.)

I believe that their direct observation of the child, added to knowledge of the meaning and usefulness of the equipment, may be one way to avoid succumbing to disproportionate levels of anxiety. This was thoroughly understood by the nurses' group when discussing the observation of Pino's first encounter with his mother:

The mother walks in, helped by a nurse, since she is still suffering from the Caesarean section. After disinfecting her hands, she hesitates for a moment, then she takes his hand, and speaks a few words to him, but does not touch him any more. She prefers to address herself to me, probably mistaking me for the doctor, and asks about her child: how much he weighs, whether he is too little, whether he will gain some weight before going home, etc. When I invite her to caress him, she says she is afraid of touching him, as if he would break.

Meanwhile, Pino opens his eyes, as though he wanted to see what is happening and who is touching him. His mother becomes a bit more confident and softly strokes his legs; she touches his feet, especially the right one, which is bandaged owing to heel-pricks; she observes his fingers and remarks on how long they are. [Observer: G. Odone]

The observation highlights two main features: (1) the mother's difficulty in approaching her child, seen in her slow progressive physical contact with him (like that described by Klaus & Kennell, 1970); (2) the mother's need to relate to her child through direct infant observation and knowledge of the main clinical parameters.

I usually try to meet the mother a few hours after childbirth, and often I talk also to the father, who is probably near his wife. I listen to the parents, who usually do not say much at this point, owing to their worry about their child. I tell them what I have seen of the child and inform them about the importance of their presence near the incubator. I also make known the times and days of the week when they can meet me near their child's incubator.

Following this, I check what is known of the parents' psychological situation and consider the emotional impact on them of the birth of a child in danger of not surviving. The assessment of the social environment to which the child belongs is important for its prognosis, but the consideration of the psychological risk faced by the parents is even more important.

I find it very useful to carry out this evaluation together with the nurses. Being with the child all the time, they have a more complete picture of the family situation than I could have at this early stage, so they provide me with information that is very useful to my intervention with the parents. I discuss with them the parents' attitudes and the frequency of their visits to the child. In the light of this background information I consider the social problems that might prevent the couple from being sufficiently present and close to their child. It may be, for example, that the parents' difficulty in being near their child's incubator derives primarily from social reasons (transport difficulties if they do not own a car; heavy family commitments, lack of baby-sitters, compelling work commitments, broken families, etc.); or it may derive from psychological problems.

The studies of Klaus and Kennell (1970, 1971, 1983a, 1983b) are a milestone in the understanding of the many aspects that are relevant to the newborn in an intensive care unit—parents, staff, and child. They stress the significance of early contact between newborn and parents. The longer this is delayed, the more disturbed will the relationship be, with very serious consequences for the child and family environment. It can happen that even when parents are emotionally ready to accept the seriously impaired child, they are prevented for social reasons from coming close to it, and psychological difficulties may arise, undermining their future relationship with the child. In situations like this we do our best to help the parents, and on my own part I try to adjust to their commitments, meeting them at the times of day when they are able to be present with their child. I behave in the same way with parents who show clear psychological difficulties in approaching their child. But if I notice that in spite of my efforts they come up with various excuses for not attending the meetings, then I give them precise appointments.

In socially and psychologically less favourable situations the method of intervention remains the same. As stated, I try to accommodate the parents' needs and adjust to the times of their visits; in return, I require greater collaboration from them, to establish a closer relationship with the child.

At this point, it may be useful to provide an example of how the first interviews have been carried out, in cases where the child is still in a critical condition regarding survival, and at risk from possible neurological sequelae.

The following intervention concerns the parents of Elisabetta, born during the 26th week, the second child after a 4-year-old sister:

Elisabetta.   Birth weight 700 g. Placenta 250 g. APGAR 4–6. Serious breathing deficiency is present. The child looks vital at birth; grasp and uncoordinated limb movements are present. Muscular tone is fair. Her trachea is intubated through the mouth in the delivery room. Some spontaneous breathing actions are present. Oxygenation is good. When she is 2 days old, she fights the respirator and shows some tremors that make it necessary to soothe her. She is given a sedative and adjusts herself to the respirator. When she is 4 days old, she appears soothed; spontaneous breathing actions are absent, thorax expansion is symmetrical. I carry out my first observation session on the same day; the nurses tell me that they have seen her parents only once. Her father seemed to be the one most upset by the sight of the girl and asked repeatedly whether she was suffering, while her mother seemed to show more optimism.

When Elisabetta is 1 week old, I ask to see her parents, but instead her rather worried grandparents turn up that day, saying that their children apologize for not being able to come and would like to know from the paediatrician about the girl's health. When I carry out the next observation, the girl is 11 days old, and I hear that the parents have not shown up yet.

When Elisabetta is 14 days old (equivalent to 28 weeks of gestation), I finally meet the parents for the first interview:

When I arrive at the department, they are already there, near the incubator. They are both very young and have gentle manners. The girl's tracheal tube has been changed today; it brings the ala of her nose up somewhat, and thus her delicate and regular profile is rather deformed. She sleeps supine, her little arms half bent near her head, her hands covered by small blue cloth gloves. Her little mouth is half open, her head is turned to the right, her right foot is touching the sheet with extended leg, her left leg is up and bent at a right angle to the bottom of the cot, the sole of her foot is leaning fully on the sheet. She moves her right leg, then she is quiet again; she moves her four limbs, then is quiet again. I introduce the girl to her parents, stressing the vitality she has shown up to now and the importance for these children of their parents' presence near them. The mother says: "I don't know what it means, but when we got near the incubator her whole body was moving." The father tells me about their "frightening" experience, but he is soon interrupted by the mother: on the 25th of December she had some brown leakage and was advised to have an emergency check; she was prescribed Miolene, but cramps persisted, and after one week she had to be hospitalized. In spite of the treatment, she still had cramps during hospitalization and, when an infection at placental level was detected, the doctors decided to just take care of her and forget about the baby. But she hoped, still hoped, the baby was still alive. The day before delivery, she felt the baby go down; she opened her legs and asked her husband to "look at what's going on". But here he said: "I saw nothing."

Her little girl, near us, is still quiet; then, assuming a serious and angry expression, she moves her whole body, gathering her limbs then releasing them outwards again. I remark that Elisabetta is a beautiful name. The mother reacts, saying with satisfaction that her eldest girl's name is Chiara, implying that this is also a beautiful name. The parents tell me that they are also worried about her: she is 4 years old and has already asked them whether they are going to love her as well. Both parents desired this pregnancy, since they wanted a little brother for their eldest daughter, in order to have a better family mix. They were not disappointed when a second girl was born, though perhaps the father's parents were disappointed, since they are from Benevento: both of their sons have girls. I point out the little girl's beauty, the delicacy of her features; the mother says she notices these things now. After delivery the mother was still very upset by that experience, and when she came to the department, she was looking for her daughter amongst the bigger babies; she only noticed the beauty of her little feet. I point out her feet, her hands—even though they are now covered by her gloves—and her features, even if, I add, the tube lifts up her nostrils too much. Then I point out the delicacy of her ears. The mother in particular appears to agree with me and seems pleased at my description, even if she again interrupts me to let me understand that her eldest daughter, who is at home, is also very beautiful.

The little girl shakes her tummy, moves her limbs, bends again. Her parents, particularly the mother, asks why. These are movements typical of sleep, I say, adding that they already show her to be very active mentally. Her parents ask me whether she is exposed to risks. I reply that so far the girl has proved to be full of vitality; the risk mainly relates to her lungs; but this can only be known with time. Once more I observe the girl: I remark that her right foot is touching the bed sheet; her mother remarks that her left foot is grasping the little tube. I say that she is evidently seeking a contact and that I had already noticed it in a previous observation; her mother says that it may be due to the fact that she used to touch the girl through her abdomen: "I also had my husband touch her, we were happy she was alive." I add that it is also important to prepare for her a recorded tape, with sounds, verbal messages, or whatever they like her to hear; this will be placed in the incubator should the girl appear to be restless and show a desire for company. Her mother asks when she is going to be allowed to touch her; I say that it is a good idea, even though only for a few moments, for now. At present, Elisabetta looks more like wishing to be left alone; we noticed, I also add, that after the first two or three days, during which she seemed more restless, she has shown herself able to quieten down, sleeping a lot; also, the nurses put a positive interpretation on her feeling at ease in the dirt when she defecates and urinates, as though she "didn't care a straw", since she was so determined to feel well. Her mother seems pleased by this description, whereas her father asks me if I think the girl has suffered particularly. I reply that as far as Elisabetta is concerned I had not noticed any particular signs of suffering. We then talk about the best times for the mother to come here, also bearing in mind the present condition of her health. In fact, her father seems to put forward a thousand problems about her coming for the time being— such as the other girl, and how even this morning (although it is a Sunday) he had difficulty coming here because he was responsible for the village's evangelic community. He then tells me that a certain type of feeding directly through the umbilical cord is practised at Monza's hospital. I reply that Elisabetta's present condition allows the use of naso-jejeunal feeding, and I explain its features.

The above observation shows the parents' difficulty in approaching their daughter: as the nurses had already noticed, the father seems to be the most inhibited. The mother, in fact, added to my comments about the girl's vitality, appearing immediately to be able to get in touch with her: "I don't know what it means, but when we got near the incubator her whole body was moving." The father, however, is not yet able to do so; he recalls, instead, the traumatic experience he had recently had. At this point even the mother feels the need to recall it— allowing us to understand, however, that she never allowed herself to be completely swept away by despair; she always hoped that the girl would still be alive. When commenting on the beauty of the girl's name, she again shows good contact with her, even though she introduces the problem of the elder girl at home (who also has a beautiful name and also needs her), so expressing her worry of tying herself down too much and letting herself become too involved with this new girl.

The mother, therefore, seems afraid of too definite a bond with a baby who is still in danger of not surviving, lest she be confronted with too deep a pain. Whereas from the comments regarding the father's parents it is possible to see that even if some worry exists about their acceptance of the child, this does not involve the mother but only the father—in fact, only the father's parents who were expecting something very different. This feeling does not appear to be destructive or dangerous for the mother or her relationship with her husband: it is not impending, it is kept away, at Benevento.

In my intervention, whenever possible, I deem it important to stop and describe to parents the beauty and delicacy of the little patient's figure. I have already hinted how significant it is for these mothers to live the aesthetic experience with their newborn as early as possible, and how they are seriously hindered from doing so. Thus achieving this experience was also difficult for Elisabetta's mother, who, as she came into the department, was looking for her amongst the biggest babies, and at first was only able to see the beauty of her feet. Here again it is possible to perceive the fear of committing herself too closely to the baby: Chiara at home is very beautiful too, while Elisabetta is still in a dangerous situation: what shall I have to face if I grow too fond of her, what if she dies . . . ?

Interrupted pregnancy

Observing her little girl enabled this mother to re-establish a lively contact with the child. She noticed her little foot grasping the tube and associated the baby's desire for contact with her husband's and her own caresses through the abdomen. In this way she demonstrated that she perceived Elisabetta as alive, lively, but still inside herself. The problem of the interrupted pregnancy was painfully and deeply felt by the parents. Mankind's struggle with life and death emerges every time human beings are faced with the existential choice of accepting the limitations of their own life cycle, or overcoming it through their children's biological and mental survival. Thus, one of the questions inherent in procreation is that of denial of or overcoming one's individual death. That is why death is always latently present in every life project. Death is also present in the delivery room and, after remaining more or less latent during the last part of pregnancy, gives rise to an anxiety that can be sensed in all the protagonists on the scene of childbirth.

Plutarch (cited in Peiper, 1961) says: "Nothing is so incomplete, nothing so needy, nothing so naked and dirty as man, when he comes from his mother's womb. Bespattered with blood, full of filth, more like a murdered than a born creature, he enters the light, so that only those in whom love is imprinted by nature can touch him, kiss him and take him in their arms" (p. 8)

In the dreams and phantasies related to childbirth, anxieties about loss, emptying, punishment, and castration, as well as anxieties related to one's child's or one's own death emerge. Concerning the embryo at the beginning of pregnancy, whatever the viewpoint (whether biological or the relational one described by Kellerhals and Pasini, 1977), its own existence is inseparable from the image of death. Extremely positive feelings, linked to a sensation of fullness and vitality from the successful conception, coexist together with deep anxieties deriving from the persecutory phantasies related the feelings of guilt of early childhood (the Oedipus complex) and to the embryo's parasitic and devouring image, which belongs to the relationship with the pregenital archaic mother.

In the event of an interrupted pregnancy, positive elements deriving from the state of pregnancy disappear, giving rise to an experience of death related to that part of oneself which is identified with the foetus itself and its content of creativity and a vital future. A deep sense of sorrow emerges also for no longer being able to raise one's child inside oneself.

The preterm newborn can, in its turn, be the object of intensely persecutory projections, which impinge negatively on the mother's mental state. During the first interview with the mother of a little girl born at 25 weeks, weighing 800 g, she asked me whether medicine had yet discovered a method for reinserting the preterm baby inside the mother's womb, so that pregnancy could continue to term. Furthermore, as if to confirm this phantasy, she told me during a subsequent interview that she hoped to become pregnant again as soon as possible so that she could give a brother to her little girl. And the mother of Stefania, a girl born at 26 weeks, weighing 680 g, described her experience in this way: "When I was admitted to hospital fifteen days before Stefania's birth, my belly did not show yet. I came out of hospital without belly and without child."

Several more examples of this kind could be given. But now I would like to go back to Elisabetta's session. The idea of asking the parents to record a tape to be put inside the little girl's incubator is a way of letting them feel closer to their child even when she is in hospital in a state of forced isolation, totally dependent on machines and people outside her familiar environment. It can give them the chance to feel a unique, intimate, direct, and unmediated bond with the baby. It is interesting to note how two sessions after this one the father asked me what they were supposed to record on the tape. When I answered that they could record anything they wished, the mother soon intervened, as though she were thinking aloud: "I don't know why it's different: if I imagine Elisabetta inside me I feel like thinking and talking to her, but now she is outside. . . ." This consideration is, in a certain way, very interesting and shows that the intervention contact with parents is useful to help the mother think about the premature birth (Berrini & Carati, 1982). (The same consideration applies to the mother's comments on the various stages of Giacomo's development in chapter three.)

It is interesting that during this stage of hospitalization mothers prefer to record songs and music that they like and used to listen to during their pregnancy. In this way they show they imagine their baby as still "inside". But when the baby's tubes are removed and it weighs over 1.5 kg and is in a sufficiently safe condition, mothers often spontaneously bring a music-box to be hung inside the incubator; the baby is no longer "inside" them; it is born and therefore needs a toy, the kind of music suitable for a born child. It is also common at this time for parents to tell me they have started thinking again about the baby's room, the cradle, and preparations for coming home. Sometimes they tell me, with evident relief, that at the weekend, for the first time in a long while, they have gone out shopping together to buy clothes for their baby.

Going back to the session with Elisabetta at 28 weeks, it can be seen that the mother was already anxious to fondle her baby and appeared pleased to hear her described as a girl who, in order to feel well, did not "care a straw" about being dirty. The same did not apply to the father, who still preferred to stay away from the relationship (he had so many engagements, he could not come often to see her); on the other hand, he believed that the baby was suffering too much, was too fragile: she could not make it "outside". He would rather she were still in the womb—mentioning the other type of feeding "directly through the umbilical cord" being used at Monza's hospital.

We can see from the material that has been presented that it seems to be very important not only to show the parents one's ability to think about the baby's somatic characteristics—its emotional, neuromotor, and behavioural patterns—but also to prove to them that one is well informed about all the other aspects of its health care, including the type of treatment used. In this way the parents can feel that their child in its entirety is present in my mind. The introduction of this new approach was not intended to replace but rather to integrate the sessions offered to parents which were previously mentioned. In cases where a seriously premature birth is a highly traumatic experience, it seems necessary to offer both kinds of intervention.

The separation–individuation process

At this point, however, what seems to be important is that the parents themselves should ask for a session in order to speak about their own, and their other children's, personal emotional situation (Box 1). Approaching them primarily through baby observation seems to allow a distinction to be made between the newborn with its pain and themselves with their personal emotional difficulty stemming from the distressing experience of a premature birth. The improved understanding by the parents of the emotions that relate to them, distinguishing them from the baby, is very important for carrying out the separation–individuation process, which is so difficult to achieve for all newborns undergoing this experience and particularly for those who will develop symptoms of cerebral palsy.

All of the mothers and two of the fathers of the babies with a birth-weight of under 900 g with whom I used this approach also requested sessions for themselves.

Here is Elisabetta's mother's session—the baby is now 27 days old:

When I enter the department at 10 o'clock, I find the mother standing in the corridor; she says that she is there because the baby's endotracheal tube must be changed. She is apparently quiet and serene; I show her into the

BOX 1
The intense jealousy problem of the elder child

When the newborn is still in a critical condition, parents frequently ask for a separate session, to talk about the problem of the intense jealousy shown by their elder child, with which they do not know how to cope. The parents are hampered by deep feelings of impotence and inadequacy, which derive from their sense of guilt. The guilt is linked not only to the newborn, who may be seriously preterm or at high risk, but also to the fact that, especially at the beginning, their elder child does not receive the attention and care he had before the new baby's birth.

It seems to me also that this can be a type of defence mechanism, enabling parents to distance themselves and not face directly the more painful and devastating sense of guilt deriving from the recent birth of the seriously preterm baby.

This problem may also be noticed in the clinical material already presented about Elisabetta—in particular in the preliminary draft of the first interview with her parents. The references to the elder daughter are numerous, and the parents' worry about not being able to give her the necessary care and affection is explicit. ("Chiara's four years old and she's already asked us if we'll still love her . . .").

small kitchen. As a matter of fact there is a great deal of activity going on in Elisabetta's cubicle, and a lot of people near her. There is an atmosphere of nervousness, and I notice that the doctor changing the little tube is not one of the most experienced to be performing this operation on such a young baby.

I close the door of the kitchen, and once the mother is seated I ask her whether she would like to look at a magazine. She replies she would rather talk. I sit in front of her, and she immediately begins her story.

She tells me she is worried because she has recently been

feeling "light-headed"; she has difficulty in concentrating, her eyes are heavy. "I am calm but cannot concentrate on housework. I have had this feeling since I left the hospital. I was there for twelve days before delivery and four days after the baby was born. I started feeling like this two days after I had come home. I believe it to be connected first of all with the pain I felt, and then with the sedatives I took. I told the doctor I had come to have these troubles explained and that I felt doped—I am becoming senile. . . . I'll give you an example: a cleaning lady comes regularly to the flat below mine and cleans the stairs, and I know her very well. One morning I went to the baker's, and he addressed me as 'the mother of that baby who was so small when she was born' (the whole village knows and talks about it). A woman behind me said that she knew about it too; I turned and asked her how she knew, and she replied that she knew me: 'I can't believe you don't recognize me, I am the person who cleans the stairs in the building where you live.'"

"I usually carry out all our household business—for my husband as well—but now I am worried, I am afraid of muddling it up. The bank manager explained something to me yesterday, but I didn't understand it."

At this point I say to her that this trouble of hers is understandable and that it is linked with the traumatic experience of such a premature birth. She continues:

"My husband is sad because the girl has no expression. . . . I believe I got rid of my problems by transferring them into the baby." I reply that, on the contrary, by delivering her baby so early she has allowed it to survive, which would not have been possible if it had been kept inside her any longer.

The mother listens with interest but goes on: "When I see her with the tubes—but she won't remember . . . does she understand what they are doing to her?" I reply that I understand her worry; these are painful experiences, from which, however, the child will later be able to recover with the help of her parents and with that of the people working in this department, who also pay much attention to those aspects.

The mother goes on talking of her problems of "light-headedness": "It is as if I were suspended; I find it difficult to do my housework. You see, you know my husband is responsible for a community: well, he often has a lot of people for dinner, and I take care of everything personally, it doesn't feel like hard work. My mother-in-law and my sister, who had come to see my daughter, had dinner with us yesterday: there were only five of us, but I had to ask my sister to do everything—I couldn't remember what to do. I am the type of person who feels sick seeing other people in pain. I know the doctors are very experienced and that Elisabetta is alright; I wasn't calm during the first few days, but I am now. The nurses have asked me if I want to talk to the paediatricians, but I don't mind, I am confident anyway.

"I was very upset by what a nurse told me two days ago—she is the one who has a nose like mine, who wears glasses and has curly hair" (I immediately single her out, the description being very accurate). "I was near Elisabetta when I noticed that the baby near her, who was so ill during the past few days, was smiling, and I told the nurse: 'She's smiling.' The nurse replied: 'It's forbidden to look at other people's children.' I was very disappointed: I am in here too, and I don't just look at my baby. I realized that that baby was very ill during the last few days; she is beautiful, but one could see she was yellow. I could never do this work." I say that the nurse probably replied like that because she was worried about the treatment the child was being given, and this might have prompted her to give such an unsympathetic response.

She tells me, at this point, that Nurse Lucia is giving her a lot of courage, and that the head nurse has been showing her around the department and also allowing her to look at the other children. "My parents were there two months

ago, in the intensive care unit, because they had eaten
poisonous mushrooms, *Ammanita phalloides*" (she
mispronounces the word) "that my father had picked.
Downstairs they were refusing to believe him because that
mushroom is very poisonous, lethal. The casualty
department at the Zingonia hospital phoned Milan and
then Bergamo and were told that my parents should come
here since both hospitals were in touch with this centre.
They are very clever. My parents felt very comfortable
here: Mummy went home after five days, Daddy after eight
because he has liver trouble. I am confident; I like reading,
and I check on what you tell me, and everything
corresponds. . . . The nurses allowed me to touch
Elisabetta again, twice—not this morning, because she
was restless. I asked the nurses what it meant, and they
replied that she is trying to breathe on her own." I confirm
this and tell her that this has been noticed from the first
few days. "I don't ask, I am confident, this is important
work. I have been in touch with Jacopo's mother" (Jacopo
is a baby born at 25 weeks, weighing 800 g, who was
discharged shortly after Elisabetta was admitted) "and I
hope to meet her to compare our experience. I don't drive
a car and find it difficult to get transport here: my
husband takes me every other night, and anyone from my
village who knows about it and is going to Treviglio offers
me a lift—I don't trust the bus. Is one allowed to stay here
in the afternoon as well?" I nod; she goes on: "Elisabetta
has changed, she looked more rosy yesterday, more
beautiful—she looked sun-tanned, really. She was calm
yesterday; she did a wee and a poo, then she raised her
bottom and moved away—she needs to be changed more
often; do you think they will teach me and then I will be
allowed to change her?" I nod, and she goes on: "She now
weighs 770 grams; she grows and gets longer. In the
womb it is completely different—a premature delivery has
never taken place in my family; I didn't even know there
were 770-gram babies. When I came here the second time,
even the baby next to her looked small to me. When I saw
her I wasn't even very disappointed . . . of course one feels
sad. I was only there five minutes; I couldn't even stand on

my feet, I couldn't appreciate what she was like . . . my
husband was with me, and my mother was beyond the
glass. . . ."

Catastrophic anxiety and the sense of guilt

From the beginning of this observation, and also during the
preceding one when the couple appeared very composed and
gentle-mannered, one is struck by the difficulty of detecting the
presence of catastrophic anxiety in a formal interview. I noticed
how, owing to her quiet and serene appearance, the mother
was able to ignore the drama that was taking place a few steps
away from us (in fact, the baby underwent a cardiorespiratory
failure, with PO2 parameters returning only very slowly to
normal).

There is something in that state of mind, however, that
worries her, and she wants to talk to me about it. Everything is
alright, she is serene, but "her head feels light". She imputes
this state of malaise—that does not allow her to concentrate,
confuses her, and makes her afraid of doing the wrong things—
to the sedatives she was using before her baby's birth: they
make her feel "a drug addict". When I connected her malaise to
the painful experience of the premature birth which she has
split and negated, she was able to come nearer and talk of the
problem more directly: her husband is in pain, and she is prey
to a terrible sense of guilt that makes her believe she got rid of
the intense pain she experienced for many days before the
baby's birth by transferring it to the baby, who is in unspeak-
able pain now. Adopting the suggestion of nurse Lucia, who
said "all mothers show a sense of guilt, and we reassure them—
it had to take place, the baby would have died if it remained
inside", I reply at this point that, on the contrary, pushing it out
at that point had allowed the baby to live.

The problem of relieving these mothers from the pressure of
guilt, which is always present to some degree, is a very relevant
feature of our intervention. At this point the mother is able to
connect her baby's pain to her own "light head"; she is unable
to face pain—other people must take care of that; doctors are

experienced; the part of herself that could face that experience is fragile, easily frustrated; and when this part of hers, which is represented by the baby girl near hers who is recovering starts feeling better, smiling, expressing itself, it is reproached ("you're not allowed to look at other people's children!"). My interventions, intended to show her the possibility of her baby's recovery from the painful experience and also through the help provided by the people near her, allow her to get in touch with the part of herself that needs help. So she says how much she felt helped by Nurse Lucia and by the head nurse.

Moreover, by reporting her parents' resuscitation experience after ingesting very poisonous mushrooms, the mother shows us in highly dramatic terms how the parents feel about the experience of such a premature birth: it is a case of feeling death inside oneself, with the chances of survival entirely dependent on the institution. Based on her experience here, this woman shows her confidence in the people who are taking care of the problem, yet she still finds no life-oriented sources inside herself. She listens carefully and verifies what they tell her about her baby, and she agrees, but only after comparing it with books. She is glad to be helped to touch the baby, because she would not be able to do so by herself; she is still unable to produce a life-supporting contact steadily. She feels the baby is not yet born, though it is no longer inside her: "I was told that under these conditions it grows, gets taller; but it would have been different inside." In the meantime she admits that the baby is getting more and more vital, more rosy, more of a girl, less inclined to be confused with dirt. But she still does not feel able to recognize her maternal function; the poisonous experience of the premature birth is still looming over her; that is why she must still get the nurses' help to change the baby. They are better mothers—that job could never be her job—she is confident and does not need to ask questions about her baby's health. She is terribly frightened by an event that she experienced as deadly; she can only be reanimated for the time being. "To get to the hospital I don't trust public transport; I only accept lifts from people who know my situation and volunteer to take me to Treviglio."

Two days after this session the mother noted the lessening of the trouble she had described as "light-headedness", on account of which "at home, they were afraid I was going to go mad".

Conclusions

The validity of the present approach, based on two modes of intervention—sessions with parents performed through infant observation, and sessions devoted to listening to their experience—seems to be confirmed by the evolution of the cases in which it has been applied (Negri, 1988).

In Elisabetta's case, one is able to see how the parents come to see the baby more frequently after the session: the father every other day and the mother daily, even several times a day. In the session following the one that has been presented, the father told me with great excitement as soon as he saw me that he was there when Elisabetta opened her eyes: "You should have seen how she moved them!"—showing he was able to recognize her vitality. As one is able to see from the material presented, the mother has also been helped to see vital aspects in her baby, and she now seems able to keep in touch with them, although her recent experience of premature birth is still very sharp and lacerating and prevents her from recognizing her own maternal attributes—the vital parts in herself.

As already mentioned, what seems to be very significant in this type of intervention is that, when approached primarily through the observation of their very young child, these parents can learn early to distinguish between emotions pertaining to the child and emotions pertaining to themselves: emotions that are dominated by the disrupting situation of anxiety induced by the premature birth. The awareness acquired by all the mothers and also by two of the fathers, through infant observation, then motivated them to ask for a session for themselves.

Maria's mother, for instance, did not wait for me near the baby's cot, as usual, when the girl was 2 months old, but came forward to meet me in the corridor. When I asked how things were, she replied: "I am alright, I don't worry about Maria, but I still have my experience in my mind", and once again she starts vividly recalling her pregnancy, her long hospitalization in the obstetrics department, her nightmare of causing the baby to "die inside her". We were standing in the corridor; the paediatrician was also present, showing much interest in her story, and I had to interrupt her in order to have her come into the small kitchen where we could sit and be quieter, and where without disturbance she could continue to relate her experiences, which were so painful and intense.

I believe that the kind of approach adopted here is a way of helping the parents of seriously premature babies to avoid being completely overrun by anxiety and despair, and to distinguish early on those aspects of experience that concern the baby from those that belong only to themselves. This seems to be very useful in establishing that process of separation and individuation which is so difficult to achieve in newborns hospitalized in the intensive care unit and especially in those who go on to develop cerebral palsy. The deepening and widening of the meaning of such concepts as "the narcissistic wound" and "the aesthetic conflict" seemed very constructive in this sense, and the work done in this way has allowed a better comprehension of violent and destructive aspects such as death anxiety. It helps the integration processes, decreasing the pressure in parents to use projective mechanisms. Not only that, but it seems that an intervention that brings parents in touch with their own and with the child's suffering parts is also able to help them recover—through the most vital aspects manifest by the child during the observation—what is most vital inside themselves.

The approach suggested here, which is capable of helping integration and individuation processes, needs to be considered not only as a help to the parents, but also—in my experience and according to the literature (Klaus & Kennell, 1983b; Minde et al., 1978)—it seems to be reflected positively in the child. An early acknowledgement by the parents of the child's intrinsic qualities in fact helps the child to give free expression to its innate skills, which support it in its relationship with the world in the process of growth, development, and learning, for the parents of preterm newborns usually develop the phantasy that everything their child can feel and learn depends totally on their own attitudes and behaviour. Hence there is a risk of subjecting the child to a rigid and suffocating upbringing, which will unconsciously push it towards an adhesive identification.

Meeting with parents of children who die

The approach described above also applies in its essential methodology to the meeting with the parents of children who die (Kennell, Slyter, & Klaus, 1970; Solnit & Green, 1959). The meeting with the mother of Bianca—born at 27 weeks, weighing 960 g, and dead on the fourth day due to sudden cardiac arrest—is reported here as an example. I had seen the girl on the previous night, and her clinical condition was satisfactory; there was no reason to let me foresee such a sudden death.

> *Bianca's parents.*   The little girl's mother is still
> hospitalized in the obstetrics department. A nurse
> accompanies me to the six-bed room. A few mothers are in
> the room with their newborn babies in their arms or in the
> cot near the bed. Some relatives are with them. A mother
> in the last stages of pregnancy is in bed talking to a friend
> of hers. Bianca's mother is curled up in bed, under the
> blankets, with her back turned towards her room-mates
> and her face towards the glass door. Her eyes are closed; I
> believe she is sleeping, and I'd rather not disturb her, but
> as soon as the nurse softly calls her she immediately
> opens her eyes. She is curled up on her left side. I sit
> beside her and introduce myself; she stares at me with her
> intense blue eyes, which soon fill with tears. At first her
> facial expression seems static, almost bewildered; but it
> gradually becomes more mobile and lively, sweet and
> willing to communicate. She tells me that she really
> wanted this baby, that everything had been alright until
> 20 days ago, when the obstetrician had told her that the
> amniotic sac had substantially lowered and the cervix was
> already dilated. "I stayed in bed, but then the baby was

born. It is a difficult moment, too many things have happened in twenty days. I have not yet thought over and understood the events. During the first period of pregnancy I was afraid of giving birth to an abnormal child. But I was told that pregnant mothers usually have these kinds of fears. The first two days after delivery I thought I hated the baby for what had happened, but ever since last night I have been hopeful, I had become fond of her, I even touched her . . . now I have a sense of guilt for what has happened."

I tell her that it was probably necessary for the baby to be born so soon, to have a chance of survival. I tell her that I had seen her the night before, and she was fine, seemed very vital, and did not seem to be suffering. The woman starts talking again and says that the little girl weighed a lot considering her gestational age. Nurses told her they would examine the placenta as well as the baby (in the post-mortem examination). She asks me: "Why did she have the drip on her head?" I explain that this is a method of feeding and rebalancing the baby; she seems satisfied by this answer. I then add that Bianca is a nice name. The woman answers that she chose it together with her husband in the delivery room. If it had been a boy, they would have called him Franco, the name of the paternal grandfather who is now dead; they had not thought about it before, there was still so much time ahead. . . . A young man arrives and stops near the bed. The woman does not stop talking to me; she goes on and says that she wants another child. She adds that she really wants a new baby. (This is a very common desire in mothers soon after an abortion, or in the same situation as Bianca's mother.) At this point the woman seems to realize the young man is there and introduces him to me; it is her husband. He has an open face, expressing a ready but controlled emotional involvement in the situation. He remains still, as though he preferred to leave enough space for his wife's pain. The time is over; I say good-bye, and the woman tells me she will come and see me as soon as she knows something about her baby.

I met the woman on the following day in the garden of the hospital, walking very close to her husband. I asked her how she felt, and she answered that she was still suffering but that she felt better than yesterday. She told me she would eventually contact me. Yet, as is the case with most dead children's parents, she has not been in touch with me since then.

CHAPTER TWO

Work with the staff

T he work programme in our department gave me the opportunity to organize meetings with the medical and non-medical staff. I was aware of the intense emotional stress experienced by the staff in the neonatal intensive care unit. I also felt it was important for the staff to be more fully involved in the emotional aspects concerning both parents and newborns. In addition, I became aware of the interest that my role in the department aroused among the staff.

The existing literature (De Caro, Orzalesi, & Pola, 1986; Marshall & Kasman, 1980) stresses the discomfort, fatigue, and tension in the context of nursing work, which often lead to the so-called "burn-out syndrome". It is not surprising that this might be prevalent in our department when one considers that it deals with children who are at the beginning of their lives but under constant threat of death. This in itself is difficult to tolerate; but it is not all. In this unit, the medical and nursing staff deal with newborn infants who, by themselves—as the Kleinian school has already pointed out—are a source of very strong and violent emotions. Martha Harris, in particular, has highlighted the extreme complexity of the task of caring for newborns—usually both strong and vulnerable at the same time—owing to the intense and deep emotions that they arouse. Therefore, if the hospital staff cannot or do not receive any help in understanding the deep emotional stress aroused by these factors, they will be more susceptible to the tiring and stressful aspects of their work, which can ultimately lead to burn-out.

Fatigue is linked to the routine and repetitive aspects of their work—namely, procedures that must be repeated over and over again within the same shift, often traumatic and invasive procedures (i.e. intubation, tube-feeding, bronchial suctioning, the taking of blood, perfusions, etc.), causing suffering for the patients who receive them and requiring great care by those who perform them. The work is made even more difficult by the problems that emerge in the relationships with the parents, who are present in the department, and problems within the institution itself.

I personally felt the need to know each one of the staff better and to know more about their specific tasks within the unit. It was difficult to arrange regular meetings, because nurses' shifts had to be taken into account and also because it was important not to burden the nurses further by requiring them to spend extra working hours in the department. This problem seemed insurmountable to me at first, probably because I was afraid of facing a new job with a group in which there were so many emotional components.

In order to overcome the above-mentioned difficulties, I thought I could arrange weekly meetings with the staff present in the department at 11 o'clock, after the neuropsychological evaluation of children prior to their discharge from hospital. The time was chosen by the nurses; it was a "relatively calm moment". I eventually had the opportunity to meet all the nurses working in the department, through the regular rotation of the shifts. A few doctors, as well as the head physician, two out of three of the head physician's assistants, one assistant doctor, the physiotherapist, a future infant neuropsychiatry specialist, and a medical student participated in these meetings on quite a regular basis.

Work method and level

The weekly meetings started in December 1982. They included discussions on free topics, reading, and comments related to the child observation sessions and to the meetings with parents.

Over the last seven years, these meetings with the staff have been held in the room where the incubator with the most seriously premature newborn is located. The group sits around the young patient and operates as a group observing the newborn inside the incubator, with "doors open", thus acting as an observing group rather than as a training group. The number of participants varies from six to nine. During the meeting some of them may leave the room to carry out their tasks.

I play the role of leader. I do not make any interpretations or give any direct advice to the group. But, in carrying out my task, I always bear in mind the objective of the meeting: namely, the deepening of our knowledge of the problems related to the young patients, in order to care for them more effectively. The work is carried out as a discussion group on the problems related to giving assistance (Bion Talamo, 1989). It is based on my training experience, acquired in the field of infant observation (Bick, 1964), in particular with Martha Harris and Donald Meltzer (Harris, 1976, 1978; Meltzer & Harris, 1985; Negri, 1989a, 1989b; Negri, Guareschi Cazzullo, et al., 1990).

I found that as in infant observation discussion groups (Vallino Macciò et al., 1990), in order for the work to develop, the staff needed to go through various mental states, which could be viewed as "typical phases": the emotional atmosphere; role neutrality; mirror resonance; and thinking about the work group. Furthermore, when tackling the problem of psychic suffering and anxiety change, I have considered the dynamic and geographic point of view, as described by Meltzer and Harris (1983).

Model evolution

The basis for this progressed from the use of a data card to infant observation work around the incubator.

Problems to be tackled

The most meaningful psychological aspects and problems inherent in the activities of people working in the intensive neonatal pathology section emerged after the first meetings with the staff. In particular, they became evident during a meeting aimed at evaluating the effectiveness of an observation card relating to young patients and their parents, which was to be filled in by the nursing staff. It was intended as a way of encouraging reflection and enabling the staff to understand the emotional problems of patients and parents (Table 3).

The discussion about filling in the card showed that it was felt as an intolerable and excessive task: "It has not yet become part of our routine work; the head nurse should say it." I noticed that nurses left to doctors the task of filling in most of the forms. Next, during the meeting, it became evident that the group's interest was mainly aroused by the case of a mother who was hospitalized in our department together with her child and who was harshly criticized and defined as "paranoid". She "would always ask everybody the same things, would not listen to others, act as if nothing had happened, and kept staring at the nurses with her swollen eyes". The harsh criticism, the anger and dislike expressed by the group towards this "paranoid" mother, who was unhappy and unable to take care of her child and who was never satisfied with the nurses' answers, made me think that in the framework of my job with the group it was essential to find a space for discussing the "paranoid mother" phenomenon. The "paranoid mother" stood for the nurses' own feelings and emotions, which were difficult to express and contain.

During this meeting I could also see that the nurses were especially annoyed by several questions asked them by parents. That is why, during the meeting, I decided to come up with specific questions related to their assistance work, in order to substantiate the idea that questions are a necessary part of a mutual exploration process. After having identified the nurses' profound interest in the questions I formulated, I hoped to demonstrate to them how the parents' "several questions" should not be interpreted as a sign of aggressiveness. This assessment of the problem has enabled nurses to develop a more empathic and ready attitude towards the parents (Box 2).

Table 3

Surname   Name   Pregnancy weeks

Admitted on   Born on   Weight

due to   at

discharged on

Mother: age   profession

Father: age   profession

Siblings:

Economic conditions: precarious

                            sufficient

                            good

                            very good

Meeting   with the mother: date
               and/or
               with the father: date

Mother's and father's visits: daily (1–2–3 times)

                            frequent (every 2 or 3 days)

                            *occasional

                            *very rare

*probable cause

PARENTS' ATTITUDE	MOTHER	FATHER
Initial preoccupation		
Collaboration with the staff		
Persistent and evident anxiety		
Critical attitude towards the Unit staff		
Depression		
Optimism—superficiality		
Indifference		
Other (i.e., desire of the child's death, etc.)		

BOX 2

Empathic attitude to parents

*A sequence from the second part of the meeting
about the "paranoid" mother.*

Following the nurses' complaint about that lady asking too
many questions, I myself start asking the group lots of questions:

MYSELF: What kind of reactions have you faced with such an
aggressive mother?

[Nurses grumble and laugh, as though they wanted to keep
down the decided aggression aroused in them by thinking of
that mother.]

L: We have to give her orders. Ten grams of milk are important for a child. For instance, yesterday this woman was
supposed to feed her child ten grams of milk, but she
didn't want to do it. We told her it was important.

MYSELF: Why was it important?

L: The mother must not deny milk to a child who screams
incessantly because it is hungry. We had to wait for her to
leave before we could feed the baby ourselves.

MYSELF: How do you behave with mothers whose children
are in incubators?

L: They soon come into our department. When the child is in
the incubator, we encourage mothers to touch the child,
and we are very careful to ensure it doesn't get a cold.

MYSELF: How do you solve the thermoregulation problem
with preterm newborns?

M: Preterm newborns are the ones with more problems. We
use a lamb's fleece to cover them; we often take their
temperature, and special incubators are also used.

MYSELF: Can the frequent temperature-measuring disturb
them?

NURSES [almost all together]:   Oh no, we use an electrical
device to measure the transcutaneous temperature.

MYSELF: And what about children born at term? How do you
cope with the thermoregulation problem?

[The nurses answer by explaining that a special device is available to keep children born at term warm. I ask if they have noticed any special reaction in babies when they become hypothermic.]

L: Generally, no. Usually they show they are hypothermic by shivering. But Doctor R has told us that this shivering is due to the fact that they are preterm children. When babies become hyperthermic, they get nervous and cry loudly.

MYSELF: What about the feeding procedure?

M: For those who do not or cannot suck because of their illness, we now use a little naso-jejeunal tube.

MYSELF: And what did you use to do before?

M: We used a gastric tube, to be inserted every time the child needed to be fed—ten times a day.

L: The naso-jejeunal tube, which has been used since 1981, disturbs the child less; also, it can be kept in position for five days, unlike the gastric one, which had to be put in and out ten times a day and was a real aggravation; children did not tolerate it, they vomited and needed to be washed.

[Other nurses then add that, in addition, the gastric tube did not allow newborns to gain much weight.]

L: With the new tube, milk is absorbed directly by the intestine. A doctor was sent to learn how to use it—to Trieste, then to Milan to Macedonia Melloni. It is much more effective in supplying milk.

[Then I ask what they do with the little tube after five days.]

L: We replace it every five days to avoid infection. Then we do the faecal occult blood test.

MYSELF: Who positions the probes?

L: We always do it.

[M and E make their apologies, for they have to leave, to take care of two children in the department.]

[For the last three and a half years, naso-gastric feeding has again been used, as the naso-gastric tube can remain in position for a month—see chapter three, Box 18.]

Moreover, from the point of view of methodology, asking questions and trying through answering them to deepen the material presented is a very important aspect of our job, for in this way the leader identifies herself with the person who presents the experience and helps to promote internal observation and the identification with the child and the parents. As is further clarified in the section below devoted to the "emotional atmosphere", the leader must enter into the details, without confining herself to just listening; by identifying with the staff, the leader will promote the group's thinking and observation abilities.

The development of our discussion meetings demonstrated the importance of this role in providing the group with the opportunity to express its primitive and violent anxieties and feelings, so that the emotions aroused by both the suffering child and its parents could be better understood (Bender, 1981). It also became clear that more suitable ways of meeting the group's needs had to be identified. Thus I thought it was a good idea to let the nurses listen to the recorded conversations held between myself and the mothers and fathers of the hospitalized children.

The discussion about technique enabled the nursing staff to understand better some often inconsistent and irritating attitudes expressed by parents. This fostered a greater tolerance and readiness to get closer to them and encourage them to spend more time with their children and to grasp the importance of their parental role from the very beginning (Bender, 1981).

Barnett, Leiderman, Grobstein, and Klaus (1970) state that the most serious effect of the separation between mother and child is the mother's lack of confidence in establishing a relationship with her child, understanding its needs, soothing and taking care of it. W. Freud (1981) has pointed out the risk to the caring attitude of mothers when their children are admitted to the neonatal intensive care unit and they are detached from involvement in their child's care. They feel superfluous, so they visit their children less and less frequently, delegating care totally to doctors and nurses.

After listening to the account of the conversations between myself and the parents, both doctors and nurses came to understand some of the parents' attitudes better and no longer criticized them, but finally learned to offer them some words of encouragement. At the same time, I noticed that the discussion meetings enabled the group's members to talk more freely not only about their difficulties with parents, but also about their own problems.

BOX 3

*Open-door observation of the newborn
in the incubator*

As described in chapter three, I changed the approach of the work-group meetings, on the basis of experience from the first observations of Giacomo, who was almost always asleep and was described through the comments of nurses and parents. I was led to think how useful it would be if nurses had the chance to observe the personality development of every newborn more frequently and systematically. Therefore I decided to hold the weekly meetings with the staff in the actual room where the most seriously premature newborn, or the newborn at greatest risk, was located.

In this setting, participants sitting around the little patient in the incubator turn themselves from a training group into a group that is "open" to observation of the newborn.

It is not the same baby who is observed each time, but always the one at greatest risk—usually the latest admission to the department. This means that during the meetings the group may discuss and compare more than one child. The number of participants may change, but they are all people involved in child care. Sometimes the department's physiotherapist or the parents—more often the mother—also attend these sessions.

The constituents of the group are flexible, but the meeting always has a precise structure owing to being centred on the child observation. The term "open door" comes from the "open days" organized in some countries to enable parents to observe children at work in their schools.

Moreover, during the first meetings I realized how difficult it was for the hospital staff to put together technical and emotional aspects relevant to the child, especially under certain specific circumstances. For instance, they were able to recognize that the child was hypothermic from its shivering, but they were unable to recognize the pain that this manifested. This is understandable, because those who must administer highly traumatizing procedures to newborn infants (heel pricks, bronchial suctionings, probe installation, etc.) and fight for their survival at the same time find it very difficult to think about the intense feelings of anxiety aroused by the infants.

This is why it seemed useful for the group to read the observation sessions of a preterm newborn from the time of its admission to our department during our weekly meetings. This reading was originally started by a medical student and carried on subsequently by myself (see chapter three). The discussion of this material and the observation of the child in the incubator (Box 3), which were both carried out directly by nurses, proved to be the most important "direct" preventive actions for the child.

Theoretical discussion and presentation of the clinical experience

These meetings—as I have already pointed out in other works (Negri, 1990; Negri, Boccardi, et al., 1990)—highlighted the process of the group's thinking towards a mental state suitable for the understanding of the situation in question. This facilitated the development of the work whose main objective was child observation and care.

In this group thought process, four different phases can be identified, the first two being preliminary phases (Vallino Macciò et al., 1990): (1) the emotional atmosphere, (2) the neutral role, (3) mirror resonance, and (4) thinking about the work group. It has been noticed that these phenomena do not occur strictly in the above order; some aspects of the next phase may emerge when the group is still going through the previous phase. Stalemate in the thought process, which may occur during one of these phases, hinders the development of the work and incurs the risk of transforming the group into a basic assumption group (Bion, 1961).

The following description of the individual phases points out the way in which each one progresses when passing on to the next, thus showing how the development of the work becomes possible.

PHASE I

The emotional atmosphere: the state of paranoid anxiety

During the meetings with the group, it is essential to take into account the impact workers are confronted with in an atmosphere charged with violent and primitive emotions, and which often turns into a paranoid anxiety state (Box 4).

If anxiety reaches paranoid levels, it can lead to the disintegration of thought, resulting in paralysis of the group's functioning. This cannot be avoided in an environment where the presence of death is so strongly sensed.

The preliminary job consists of taking this excessive anxiety into consideration. It is therefore important to set up a group that recognizes the need to deal with these emotions. During

---

BOX 4

The emotional atmosphere

The emotional atmosphere is, by definition, a vague mental state characterized by gross, unorganized, undetermined, shapeless sensorial elements, which flow out in all possible directions. These sensations/emotions, which have been defined as "beta-elements" by Bion, are discharged externally as projective identification. Sometimes they are excessive, and the individual must free himself from them because he feels oppressed by them; at other times he wants to share this discomfort with other people.

the first meetings, the group usually tends to talk about a sense of imminent death and irreparable events. Then comments are made about one's unpreparedness and inability to face the situation. Soon the emergence of a paranoid anxiety breaks through the defences. However, there is almost always a group member who shows himself to be capable of thinking in a way that enhances his own and the other group members' ability to examine reality and to take action.

The presence of this thinking member helps the leader to point out the group's difficulties and to face the different fears that impinge on the various actions. This is the first step in untangling the situation and enabling the group to move in other directions, so that sensory, perceptive, and attentive components can re-emerge and finally allow work to continue. This is a preliminary stage in which my role as leader serves the purpose simply of alerting awareness to the fact that the intense emotional atmosphere interferes with the effectiveness of the nursing activity. As the example below shows, I let myself be permeated by the atmosphere without, however, being possessed by it. It may seem strange that apparently obvious modes of intervention are necessary. But one must bear in mind that the presence of a person who apparently plays only a passive role, merely listening, has a necessary though not often noticed function in group dynamics. This person is indeed fully active and attentive, thus allowing anxiety to be expressed without being acted out. In this way the paranoid anxieties are contained, and no persecutory ghosts take shape or become embodied in ethical biases or bizarre objects (Bion, 1967a). The leader's role is, in fact, of the utmost importance and allows a first reflection to be made, thus helping the group to find a way to get rid of all the "toxic substances" produced by a mental state disturbed and confused by anxiety.

Example. During this short session, we see how four nurses describe a situation. (It should be borne in mind, when reading the accounts of these sessions, that the people and events referred to express the thoughts and ideas of the group.) The four nurses and the physiotherapist are present at the meeting, and I relate the conversation I have had with the mother of Elisabetta,

who was prematurely born at 26 weeks, weighing 700 g,
and is still in a critical condition (the session is fully
reported in chapter one).

The nurses' comments relate to the impolite treatment of
Elisabetta's mother by one of their colleagues. The nurse
caring for another young patient had said to her: "You are
not allowed to look at other people's children" when she
had called the nurse's attention to the child in the cot next
to her own daughter, who is in a better condition. At this
point the head nurse, Piera, interrupts my reading and
comments: "How categorical we are—I would have said
yes, she's smiling. . . ." Maria, another nurse, soon
interrupts: "For a nurse it is difficult to react properly
when a child is not well: equipment does not always work
properly, the doctor cannot always be summoned
immediately, and we have to cope with our feelings, so it
may happen that at times we no longer know what is the
best way to behave."

I point out the difficulty of meeting many needs at the
same time. Maria answers: "Certainly, we must not behave
like our colleague Federica, who has shown the parents of
a child with Downs syndrome a medical book with brutal
photographs and descriptions of the disease: or who, in
reply to a father complaining about a doctor, said 'you are
absolutely right, that doctor is not at all good at medical
examinations'; or who, after taking the respirator away
from Roberto because it was needed for another young
patient, said to Roberto's parents 'you are right to be
worried because, you see, if Roberto needed the respirator
again, what would he do?', etc."

At this point I say: "I realize that your position is very
delicate and difficult; it is necessary to talk to parents, but
you cannot say everything."

The head nurse, Piera, comments: "Our position is really
difficult. We have to cope with the child's critical condition
and justify all our actions to parents, who have a right to
be involved, but only to a certain extent. There needs to be
a balance. Yet we must refrain from saying, 'this does not

work, let's try it this way or that way'. There are times
when we would prefer not to have parents around; too
much is required from us, as nurses. Not all manoeuvres
are perfect, and we need to say to each other: 'Pump, move
it, let's try this. . . .' We are as careful as possible, but we
also know that we are observed and must stay calm."

The linkages here would be difficult to understand if one did
not take into account the actual situation. I had been reporting
a conversation with the mother of a seriously preterm infant.
The head nurse's examination of another nurse's impolite attitude then gave rise to four comments on completely different
subjects.

The situation with this group was similar to one I had
encountered in another discussion group—of an infant observation within the family—where we concluded that "the examination of the error made can be a starting point for exploring
the meaning of the observed situation more thoroughly". It is
important to observe mistakes that are made under the pressure of excessive anxiety and try to understand how much
these mistakes derive from the nurses' own problems and how
much from the situation in which they find themselves. Examining this situation leads to the so-called "mirror resonance"
phenomenon inside the work group. Thus Maria re-experiences
the violence of the emotions felt by the "impolite" colleague,
who was busy taking care of the seriously ill child.

Inconclusive comments are made in consequence, thus
demonstrating a group in a "fight-and-flight" situation. Maria's
interventions seem to divert from the central issue: the discussion of the child with Downs syndrome, completely out
of context, then switches to the parents' anxiety about the
adequacy of a doctor's examination, and then to the question of
the early extubation. If the link between the nurses' phantasies
and the defence against violent (but not yet evident) premoni-
tions were missed, the leader would risk being overrun by this
basic assumption process.

The situation to which Maria reacted in such passionate
terms, of the nurse attempting to care for the seriously ill
baby and at the same time to respond to Elisabetta's

mother, suggested the following strong metaphor: "It is difficult to think when a war is going on. But the situation in our department is even more complicated, because at war there is a battle-front and a back line, and it is easy to locate the front line, whereas here the situation is much more complex; a 'multi-front' exists. You do not know what to pay attention to; pressures and stimuli bombard you from all directions, and it is not immediately possible to distinguish between the negative pressures that must be opposed and the positive stimuli that should be followed. It is difficult especially to ward off the pressure towards useless if not dangerous actions."

In other words, you must be attentive in all directions, able to discriminate, and ready to accept less than fully satisfactory results. You should face the situation initially by talking about the kind of "bombardment" to which you are exposed. War and battle metaphors are used to highlight the difficulty of the situation. Then you can start talking about it, giving it some preliminary order, making a sort of map with little signals in order to recognize the features of this situation of primeval chaos. In a situation like this we are pulled in many different directions. The difficult part is to know what you have to pay attention to, and which is the best observation point.

What can the leader do? She must intervene as moderately and as unobtrusively as possible, while containing the emotional charge of the situation, and at the same time leading the group back to the problem under question. In order to achieve this, it was important for me to bear in mind the fact that the subject of our work is the child. It was useful, for instance, while listening to the nurses during this session, to consider all the positive experiences we had shared in obtaining very satisfactory results with many other children when the overcharge of highly persecutory components seemed to have erased them. (I was helped by the memory of the positive experiences to listen and to help the group.)

The war situation conjured up in Maria's description involved a paranoid anxiety, which aroused defence mechanisms. First of all, it can be seen how my first intervention—declaring my understanding of their emotional difficulties in that specific situation—shifted the negative aspect of the parents/nurses relationship out of the way: this was projected out of the department onto the superficial colleague, who now works in another hospital. Having overcome the problem of the parents, Maria turns to that of the child and gives three examples that illustrate the defence mechanisms and their purpose. Moreover, she seems to say metaphorically that the child's survival does not depend on the nurse's care: its insufficient vitality owing to its Downs syndrome is an intrinsic factor. In this way Maria pushes away the nurses' responsibilities. The newborn is in a critical condition for genetic reasons—its Downs syndrome. The schematization, generalization, and reduction of the problem to the encyclopaedia illustrations stress its extraneous character even further. Texts also state that, at a certain age, these children are more prone to cardiopulmonary deficiencies (this is not verbalized by Maria but is implicit in the context).

At this point, the nurse takes the parents' despair into consideration, although it is immediately discharged and blamed on the ineffective doctor, who is metaphorically held responsible for the birth of the fragile Downs syndrome child. It is implied that if the doctor had warned the mother in time, things may not have gone that way.

This suggestion offers the key to the interpretation of the third phase: framed around the question, how does the birth of a scarcely vital Downs syndrome child happen at all? Its defects stem from medical causes, so such a birth must occur because of an early untimely extubation. What does untimely extubation mean in this context? It means that the mother was not correctly informed and advised by the doctor: before the age of 40 she "had done many other things"—as though this implied that she had "removed the respirator" from the child that was to be born, thus causing its Downs syndrome.

We can see how the succession of apparently inconsecutive moments described by the nurse in fact results in this defensive configuration. What is told in the first phase is then completed in the second and third ones. The reason for the child's poor vitality cannot be attributed to the limitations of the nurses' care, but only to its intrinsic Downs syndrome. The encyclopaedia schematizes and generalizes the problem exemplified by the

inefficient doctor who is incapable of performing effective examinations and who has not adequately prepared the parents—
who have made an "early extubation" of their child.

At this point, my intervention enables the head nurse to
express the difficulties verbalized by her colleague more
clearly. It is now possible to analyse the situation objectively
without resorting to any defence mechanisms. Piera plays the
role of the thinking member and introduces the concept of
the neutral role. (We recall that in her first comment at this
meeting she did not agree with her impolite colleague, saying:
"How categorical we are—I would have said yes, she's smiling.")
Piera's words sound like the group's unanimous thought. She
seems to say: "Professor Negri's orientation is interesting and
worth following, but she complicates the situation. Which are
the events that deserve our attention? What levels of experience
are we aiming to achieve? If one focuses on one particular level,
one loses other links. If one goes too far in one direction, one
can be cut off from all the rest. It is extremely difficult to find
the right balance for maintaining the ideal position, and it may
be achieved at high emotional cost: people expect too much
from us as nurses."

A precise meaningful sequence can be seen in the various
movements of the conversation in this session, which is an
indication of the commitment of the group.

PHASE II

The concept of the neutral role

The first movement in this phase consists of mourning and the
representation of anxiety; the second is founded on infant
observation and hope.

Mourning and the representation of anxiety

The work carried out by the group in an emotional situation
like the one described above enables it to relate to the subject
under discussion and tolerate the violence ensuing from the

charged emotional atmosphere. In this way the group averts the danger of being dragged into defence mechanisms, which would prevent the work from progressing through the successive phases. Then the group faces situations that arouse an increasingly intense emotional involvement. One of these is a typical feature of this working environment: namely the death of a child. When this situation is first approached, the group is riddled by excessive anxiety, which triggers defence mechanisms aimed at avoiding a sense of guilt. This is the first common reaction shown by any mourning person, and it leads to a repetitive and sterile set of complaints, accompanied by persecutory aspects. At this point, the leader's intervention is meaningful and should aim to link the emotions of the group with the question of the neutrality of the role, thereby enabling the group to understand how the role and its professionalism constitute a defence against the experience of pain. It may seem a trivial intervention, yet it is essential, in order to create a space for the initial expression of the mourning—the pain due to the loss of the baby.

The group comes to reach this stage not in a stable manner but through a whole series of ups and downs, with oscillations through which emerge both defensive intrusions and the mirror resonance phenomenon—when, through primitive projective identification processes, the nurses experience a resonance of the same emotions felt by mothers suffering for their babies. In this way they represent the anxiety and approach the pain of the death, performing the first movement in the mourning process.

Also, in sessions dealing with death or other deeply depressing subjects, some external factors always creep in unobtrusively, bringing an aura of salvation with them in the manner of the *deus ex machina* of Greek tragedy. A basic assumption group process with its characteristic emotions becomes recognizable in the group in the form of a certain mythology being played out: the story of a handicap that is eventually overcome and cured, as in stories of children seen as struggling heroes, or of the courageous mother who grants life to her little daughter (see the example of Sabrina, below). Yet, in this context, such emotions do not prevent the group from thinking; rather, they act as a light underlying ebb and flow, carrying it along. The leader must grasp and accept this atmosphere because it allows the group to nurture hope, which is the essential prerequisite for the group's progress. Unformed thought processes and oscillations emerge, which will then take shape in the following phase where, by observing the baby's most vital expressions, the nurses will leave ever more space for hope and reflections on the care of the baby.

Example. The session described here took place seven days after a previous one. Four nurses, a medical student, and a children's neuropsychiatry student were present. The baby, named Stevens, had died the day before.

As soon as she sits down, the nurse Luciana starts talking: "At 5 o'clock he was gasping for breath, there was a decrease of PO2."

The nurse Bambina adds: "Then PCO2 also dropped."

Lucia: "First, he was extubated, then excessively reintubated. He was not a strong child, not robust, unlike Elisabetta and Giacomo. Dr M says he had his duct open."

I say that I had spoken to his parents, who had shared their despair with me. His mother told me: "He died because I nurtured too many hopes." The nurse Bambina comments: "One whole month of hope." Her colleague Luciana adds: "What a pity, he was here for such a long time."

It can be seen how during the first stage of mourning the group is driven by excessive anxiety. Initial defensive behaviour appears, in the use of the specific medical terminology, to hide behind professionalism ("a drop in PO2 and PCO2, he was extubated, reintubated, open duct . . ."). The idea of death due to the PO2 drop is similar to the previously mentioned Downs syndrome child case, when the parents were shown the medical text with illustrations.

The death of a young child is an unnatural event and, therefore, unacceptable. So it can only be thought of in abstract "professional" terms. Life is seen by the nurses at this point as something analogous to respiration, which is provided by a machine and must not go below a certain level. For in this phase, to avoid an excessive sense of guilt the need arises for the nurses to resort to something external to find a justification for the child's death, such as too many intubation manoeuvres on a fragile and also probably cardiopathic child. My intervention, aimed at calling attention to the mother, enables the nurses to work out the concept of the neutral role: they no longer need to express themselves in "professional" terms, but start talking about the dead baby in a passionate way.

One month of hope is not much, but for such a small child it is a long time. They pay homage to him in this way: he was not a sufficiently strong child to be subjected to so many manipulations and intubations; yet he struggled for a long time, a whole month, and for this he deserves to be given credit. When his mother said, "he has died because I have nurtured too many hopes", it is as though she meant that her excessive hope had crushed his weak energies: the excessively strong hope is like the excessive reintubation mentioned by the nurses.

At this point the group talks firstly about parents who have taken pictures of their dead child; then about epileptic or very disturbed mothers, like Carlo's mother; then about the mother of Sabrina, a 3-year-old girl with serious kidney problems who is bound to die. This little girl has survived thanks to her mother's heroic courage. Then a nurse, referring to this lady, exclaims: "When she is not here, I love her, but when she is here I feel I hate her." One of the group members then talks about what is done in the department to help parents.

A defence mechanism can again be observed here, in the association between very young children who succeed in surviving, and their very disturbed mothers. Death is metaphorically caused by something intrinsic in the baby—such as, for instance, the patent *ductus arteriosus*—due to a very ill mother who, because of her illness, has "condemned" her child "through the malformation" even before its birth. But the group soon finds some external redeeming element. They start to talk about Sabrina's mother, the "courageous mother", who enables her already "technically" dead child to survive. A nurse says:

"When she is not here, I love here, but when she is here I feel I hate her."

Sabrina's mother stirs up strongly conflicting feelings in the group, in the same way that other highly esteemed figures do. The figure of Jesus Christ, for example, evokes a sense of admiration and emulation on the one hand, but, on the other, the excessive perfection characterizing this figure is found difficult to tolerate and becomes a source of anger. Sabrina's mother lives in an atmosphere of great idealism, which makes anyone around her feel extremely inadequate. They feel guilty and feel they must justify themselves in relation to such a courageous mother. So they describe in detail all their efforts to help the parents in the department. The lady is hated when she is present but loved when she is absent—for hate is in a dialectical relationship with love; those who love very much cannot prevent themselves from hating very much, just as the saints who loved so greatly also felt fierce hatred towards "sin", "the devil".

The atmosphere in the group has now become stimulated, elevated. Faced by the subject of death, they search for all the life-giving resources available: as in the myth of the courageous mother who ensures life for her child, and now the tenacity of the child who struggles for survival for a whole month—in Luciana's funeral oration for Stevens: "It's such a shame, he has been here for so long!" All these indicate the emergence of emotions belonging to the basic assumption group.

At this point, Lucia and Luciana start talking about the difficulty experienced by a mother when breast-feeding her infant; they talk about "cow" mothers. Luciana recalls her own experience, when she was ready to feed her child but felt depressed and worried, even though she was a nurse and the birth of her child was a normal one.

I remark on the meaningful choice of the child's name. Stevens was the name chosen by the mother for her child, and the student nurse recognized its origin in a television serial, as the name of a very fine and sensitive homosexual who is not understood by his father. Then Luciana talks about Melody, another girl with an unusual name. Lucia

said: "I did not think Stevens would have died, but the
PO2 level dropped."

Somebody knocks at the door: it is the orthopaedic doctor
intending to visit a child, but the nurses do not allow him
to enter unless he gets changed, which he refuses to do
and so leaves the room. They decide to take this up with
the paediatrician.

Meanwhile the student nurse asks me whether I am taking
care of a child with Downs syndrome who is the child of
one of her acquaintances. . . .

So nurse Luciana begins to talk about her own experience:
and, through the mirror resonance phenomenon, she re-experiences the same emotions felt by the mothers in the department,
who are worried, anxious, and depressed, even when their
babies are fine. Then they focus again on Stevens, who is so
fine and sensitive and not understood by his father: he is a
fragile child, weak, as a homosexual might be seen—a man who
lacks something, a certain virile initiative. Death comes when
life and vitality decrease (like the "PO2 drop").

At this point, it is interesting to note the effect of the orthopaedic doctor's intervention—the man who repairs only bones.
He refuses to get changed: he is concerned only with the child's
skeleton, not the rest. Thus, he becomes the metaphorical
representation of the group's thought: "Should we take care of
living children, who are partly dead owing to cerebral damage—
should these children be seen only partially, like little animals,
as the orthopaedic doctor does when he thinks only of the
skeleton and refuses to get changed? Or should we think of
them and treat them as whole human beings?" After raising
this question, the subject of death emerges again.

After the episode with the orthopaedic doctor, the group
concentrates again. Luciana says: "The dead baby stayed
there until four o'clock in the afternoon. I did not look at
it. It was difficult. . . . I have been working here for
thirteen years now; the first cases all happened to me—so
many dead children. I cried . . . then there were my
colleagues' accusations ('they all happen to you'). I cried so
much."

I say that she is a nurse who has seen the history of the whole department.

Luciana says: "You know what happened to Giusy?" (the old head nurse who opened the department and who now lives in another town). "Her husband is dying of cancer. . . ."

So many dead children! You cannot look at death, you can only put it aside. The nurse has been working here for thirteen years; she has seen so many dead children, but it is as though it were the first time, when she "cried so much". My intervention, which is intended to acknowledge the fact that she has tolerated this long mourning experience and that she is embodying the whole department's history, enables her to approach the problem and face death. She identifies herself with the old head nurse, who is now assisting her dying husband and is therefore able to take care of somebody who is dying.

Towards the end of the meeting, a nurse mentions Angela, a nurse who was prematurely born as a twin, and whose mother insisted on her daughter working here.

Hope and infant observation
with a view to taking care of the infant

Hope: It is interesting to observe the group's oscillation of thought, which starts in the first phase of mourning and the representation of anxiety. The whole process is like listening to an andante: from the adagio—which refers to dead children, who cannot be looked at—to crying for their loss and for the death of a person dear to one of the group members, and finally the ending of the movement, when one recovers, and life reappears, followed by hope.

Although this is a department in which death looms continuously, constant references are made during the meetings to other contrasting situations, which involve the utmost appreciation of life. In the example given above, this side of things was represented by the "courageous mother" with the nephropathic daughter, and ultimately by the story of the girl who had been born preterm with little vitality and who later became a nurse—someone who promotes life.

In this phase of the work, the desire for life is always sustained by someone: it may be me, or one of the parents, or a nurse who feels more confident about the survival of the little patient, or the child itself. In fact, during most of the sessions, it is above all the child who embodies the energies of the staff through its vigorous recovery and development. If we consider the dynamics of the situation, with the thought flowing from one group member to another, we can see how the generation of hope is one of the introjective functions of a family, and how it is not necessarily bound to one or both parents but can also be lodged in one of the children (Meltzer & Harris, 1983).

So, even if the nurses are aware of suffering as an intrinsic part of their job—"a job which requires the utmost commitment without knowing at all what the outcome will be"—there is now also space for hope, which in turn leads to a new way of thinking about the child. In this phase, which proves to be the most intense of all, the staff gradually construct a mosaic from descriptions of the child, which helps them to understand better the little patient's needs and emotional situation. From this, the group can develop a more specific child care pro-gramme. Most of the environmental interventions—listed in Table 2—were identified, discussed, and assessed during this phase of the group meetings.

Example. The format I am referring to in this example is that of an "open-door observation session of the newborn in the incubator". In the meeting described below, a curiosity that is different from previous meetings and a new interest in the child's mental life can be observed.

The group is now ready to face anxiety about death. They do this through their comments on Lino, a child who was born during the night at 31 weeks, weighing 1280 g.

The meeting takes place around the incubator. Monica, the nurse, says:

"At 7.30 A.M. Susanna and I were present; Luciana came later because she—fortunately!—had a cold. Lino underwent a terrible crisis. He remained black for an hour, the tube was wrongly placed, and only one lung was ventilated."

Monica and Susanna go on speaking about this episode. They say that such an experience takes ten years off your life. Monica shows her colleague the life-line in her palm: she says that it is short but crossed by the fortune line.

Thus the nurses face fear, the desire to escape, and the feeling of being robbed of years of life. Once this anxiety has been confronted, the possibility of looking at the child now emerges. Luciana approaches Lino's incubator, notes that the temperature setting is correct, and removes the sheep's fleece cover: "Let's undress him, so we can start seeing him", she says. Susanna says "he's still breathing by himself", and I comment: "What vitality!"

The optimism of my comment—intended to underline the significance of the clinical data about the child's breathing ability—is not shared by the head nurse, Piera, who makes her objection by referring to another child mentioned in other meetings (Gianluca), saying: "I am not totally confident about him." Being alive is different from being vital. Susanna, on the other hand, agrees with me, which she shows by pointing out Gianluca's various improvements and his vitality in touching the incubator walls. Monica then adds greater definition to her colleague's comment: "Gianluca always places his feet in the opening of the incubator, he grasps at the glass; he reacts more and is less listless. He has gained weight; now he is awake." At the same time she shows all the signs of the baby's outward-reaching movements.

Infant observation: "If one did not actually see these tiny children, one would not believe it", says the physiotherapist present at the meeting. Life and death are so close. The problem to be faced is, therefore, the following one: "Should one look at these tiny and vulnerable creatures, or avert one's eyes from them?" At this point the group starts talking about Andrea, a child who had been admitted to our department a few years previously and who had run the risk of dying seven or eight times during his time in hospital, but had always overcome these crises after being resuscitated. Now he still has some motor difficulties, but the nurses recognize that he is an intelligent child, able to communicate, learn, develop, and grow up.

One can see from the nature of the telling of these stories of children in the department how the group's attitude and thinking have changed since previous sessions. Learning to tolerate the death of newborn infants enables them to see other aspects as well. Both the children's suffering and their vital resources must be taken into account by the group, especially when engaged in taking care of them. The mental process oscillates here between the risk of death and then the vital recovery appearing paramount. We can understand, then, why looking at these children—which costs ten years of life—is then counterbalanced by the line of fortune (life) in Monica's phantasy.

As the various sessions develop, one can see that in observing not only the child's necessary functions, but also other intentional movements and qualitative features (which the nurses interpret in a poetic way), one can eventually obtain a more complete picture of the child; this shows that anxiety has been worked through. The pattern is as follows:

> Different nurses make comments, and Lino's mother is also present.

> "Lino is good at night. He sucks. He won't give up the dummy, even for a while."

> His mother says: "I am still slightly worried about him."

> I note how vigorously the child is sucking his dummy, and I interpret his behaviour as a sign of great vitality.

> Monica adds: "He pulls out his tubes three times a day—morning, midday, and night." Then she calls our attention to Lino's new look. She has put a sort of sweater on his little cover, as if to imagine him as an older child. She seems pleased. Then she says that the music-box put inside the incubator by his parents plays a nice lullaby, and they let him listen to it in the morning.

> Luciana adds: "We always turn it on, whenever it seems useful; it's his parents' gift for him."

In the meantime, Lino touches the incubator wall with his little hand. I call their attention to it. At the same time two nurses comment: "He's happy; it's what he likes most."

"He's good, he looks into people's eyes, he sometimes knits his brows . . . he makes grimaces like Elisabetta. He likes being bathed, touched; he pulls himself up with his little head, letting us understand that he wants to be turned. Last night he made himself heard—he wanted to be cuddled."

In the following session, the evolution of the mental process that has enabled the group to look at the infant becomes even clearer. Nurses talk about parental functioning in relation to the child's as well as their own suffering. This comes about through a story told by nurse Elena. It is the story of Lino's uncle, a disabled adult, who was living in an institute for the disabled. During an unexpected visit made by his parents to the institute, they found him dirty and neglected, so they decided to bring him back home. The group praised the high sense of responsibility shown by the parents of this disabled person. Through this I perceived the group's appreciation of the work we were doing together, which is aimed specifically at the overall well-being of the child and at enabling nurses to observe it. The nurses identify themselves with the handicapped person's parents, recognizing their ability to play a responsible parental role with regard to the distressed newborn patient. Through this identification they are able to observe and comment on the child's expressions—"He looks into people's eyes, he sometimes knits his brows, he grimaces, . . ." etc.

Infant observation
by means of the nurses' written descriptions

Following the work fostered by observation and by the experience of the "open-door observation of the newborn in the incubator", some nurses have spontaneously felt the need to write down their own profile of the seriously premature child, as observed during their work. This profile is then discussed with the group during the meetings.

The profile of Oscar, born at 27 weeks, weighing 1050 g, is given below. It was written by Serena Tomsic in collaboration with her colleague Rosanna Facchetti.

"I saw Oscar for the first time when I returned from holiday, and he was 16 days old. Even though the baby was intubated, he was very lively in his reactions. He soon aroused a deep tenderness in me. His features were regular and his cheeks rather plump, even though he only weighed 1.050 kg.

He was greatly disturbed by the naso-tracheal tube. He initially opposed the respirator and did not like being fondled, especially on his little head (owing to the intravenous drip being repositioned). He was extubated when he was 18 days old. On the doctor's instructions, intranasal probes were put in, but he never tolerated them—he always tried to pull them off with his hands, head, or legs, moving them upwards or downwards in the cot. That was why we were obliged to position the probes better, using little sand bags to keep his head turned in a certain direction. Oscar was very nervous and irritable.

When he was only 20 days old, following the doctor's instructions, the O2 supply device was applied, because the child did not tolerate the intranasal probes. Thanks to this, he became calmer, because it was possible for us to change his position more often.

From that morning, the baby began to show his preference for a certain position. We noticed that he got nervous and irritable when lying supine and was calmer when prone. From watching him, we came to the following conclusions about his behaviour:

• He wants his hands to be left free from gloves, so he can touch the things surrounding him in his cot (especially the naso-gastric feeding probe, which he often grabs with his hands).

- He touches the edges of the cot with his feet, and he loves them being stroked and kissed, even though he is ticklish.

- He is annoyed by light and shows it by closing his eyes when a light source is directed towards him.

- He loves listening to any kind of music (heart beat, or even the radio).

- He loves sucking not only the dummy (which is too big for him and after a while always slips out of his mouth), but also the edges of the O2 mask, or the piece of gauze soaked in sweetened water.

- Starting on the 25th day, the child has had some bradycardiac crises, which will eventually be overcome spontaneously or owing to stimulation. For this reason, since he was a month old, we have positioned him on a water mattress. We noticed that the bradycardia crises largely subsided and the child became calmer and had an air of well-being when the water mattress was rocked.

- He seems to show interest when people talk to him or when he is stimulated (nappy or posture change), and he shows it by opening his eyes.

PHASE III

Mirror resonance:
nurses experience mothers' and children's feelings

As already mentioned, the "mirror resonance" is a phenomenon that occurs regularly during meetings of the group, and refers to the realistic projective identification that develops with the individual's social awareness (Bion, 1967a; Bion Talamo, 1989; Klein, 1955; Vallino Macciò et al., 1990). It is an early identification in the sense of being fragile and superficial, as can be seen by the way in which the group easily passes from one identification to another.

This phenomenon is determined by the particularly intense emotional stress caused by events in the department. It leads to the creation of a group situation in which nurses live the emotional experiences of parents and children. This mental process of projective identification is a necessary and unavoidable step in the group's thought dynamics. The group can achieve a full understanding of the emotions involved only when it experiences them, living through the suffering and interaction of mother and child. The group leader needs to take mirror resonance into account, pointing out to nurses that they are experiencing an unconscious identification with parents and child. In this way the group can focus on the intensity of the anxiety and the emotional conflicts within the relationship, and so can understand the enactment of defence mechanisms. The group is thus able to find words to think about the feelings of the children and parents, and to show their concern and empathy for them.

In addition, this process leads to further development in the work, by motivating the nurses to reflect on their own emotional reactions and to assess them not only in relation to their own behaviour and feelings towards parents and children, but also in relation to themselves and the doctors within their work group. This leads them to consider the significance of the group and to realize the importance of protecting it from destructive attacks. They recognize that the group is the prerequisite for the continuation and development of their work.

> *Example:*   This session, which takes place three weeks after the one described previously, seems quite unusual. Nurses Bambina, Monica, and Angela, together with the physiotherapist, Donatella, are present.

> Bambina soon comments: "There's something I would like to understand. There was a 30-year-old mother, whose newborn child had nothing seriously wrong; she was quite experienced, because she had other children at home, and she expressed herself using the appropriate technical terms—like 'stenosis' etc.; she had milk, everything was alright; but when it was time to go home, she came up with all sorts of excuses, saying that her breast was

swollen, and so on and so forth, because she did not want to leave. It took two hours to persuade her to go."

I comment that here mothers feel protected and supported.

Monica says: "Giorgio's mother—the baby who always vomited—always asked for drops for her child, then she was quiet."

The beginning of the meeting is unusual: the nurse indicates that in this department of seriously ill patients there is also a mother who is aware of the fact that there is nothing seriously wrong with her child, a mother who can use technical terms and who has enough milk to feed her child. Why is she there? Why does the nurse talk about her? Bambina seems to say, on the one hand, "What is a mother with so much milk, culture, experience, doing there? She is occupying a place that should be left to other mothers who really need it." On the other hand, she is also trying to express something else—namely, her desire for other mothers and children of the department to be in this same situation. It is as though she wanted to say: "If this were the situation, we nurses would not feel so sad and despairing." Soon afterwards the group starts talking about the vomiting child, as though they wanted to vomit away such an "unimportant" situation, so as to make room for children in greater need—or, alternatively, as though they wanted to vomit and get rid of all these seriously ill children, because they should all like to be the one with only minor problems. They seemed to want to rub away the extremes, the contrast between minor and serious cases, thus expelling the element that creates unpleasant comparisons. My intervention tries to call the group's attention to the function of the department. This is like our work group—a place that offers protection, like an unbiased parent who is ready to welcome everybody, a life-sustaining machine. As the session continues, the meaning of the intervention becomes clearer:

Bambina adds: "That mother talked so much, she did not seem shy, she talked a lot, she hid her fear."

I refer again to the department's protective function for these parents, and I recall Yuri's mother, who even after her child's discharge always came here to ask for advice. I then add how a vomiting child is always a cause of concern for the mother, and how we in the group are reliving their feelings.

Monica says: "I am not worried about vomiting; I feel well when I vomit. In this case the mother is particularly worried that the child vomits after she has fed it herself, whereas when we feed it, everything is alright."

Careful examination of the features of this discussion gives us a deeper understanding of what is going on. We see how the 30-year-old mother (the same age as Nurse Bambina), who is apparently well-prepared and self-confident, expressing herself in technical terms, stands for one of the nurses. "Mirror reso- nance" is taking place here, enabling the group to share the feelings of the mothers. It is as though Bambina wanted to say: "There are those who do not have serious problems, but are afraid, like the mother who seemed so well prepared and edu- cated but did not want to leave. Everything is not what it appears to be: when a person does not show any particular problems, it does not necessarily mean he does not have any. The full breast conceals something that is not evident but must not be ignored. There is a need for protection and support— such as the department can offer for parents and children, or the group can offer for us, the nurses." Monica's comment then clarifies Bambina's one, stressing how problems are not the same for everybody. Identifying herself with the vomiting child, she tells us that she feels well when she vomits. In this way she implies that the child does not necessarily reflect the mother's feelings. It has its own personality, which may make it feel well despite the violent action of vomiting, although its mother experiences this as alarming.

Monica also seems to say: "There are things that are not so meaningful but that may be vomited out." Reflecting on the child who vomits not because of gastric problems but because of a psychic one, she brings the group's attention back to the mother. It is the mother who is afraid, and it is implicitly recognized that the psychic problem belongs to her and needs to be digested. The child does not vomit after being fed by the nurse, because there is not such a deep emotional involvement.

The session continues. Nurse Angela comments: "It's strange. Carlo's mother seemed to have no problem at all . . ."; Bambina adds: "She went on talking and talking, asking me silly questions." Donatella, the physiotherapist, says: "She told me she wanted to go to the mountains at Christmas." Monica says: "She didn't like talking about herself. She had had a child who was born dead, who she never talked about. When it was necessary to go to Bergamo for the child's brain scan, she did not want to go. When the doctors saw the pictures, they were rather alarmed and worried. . . ."

I say that the mother is trying to defend herself from deep anxieties.

The members of the group want to communicate that their relationship with the child is only possible if they consider the problem in depth: namely, learn how to face death, "perform the brain echography" in order to know more, understand and appreciate all the child's characteristics, even the slightest and least obtrusive ones.

PHASE IV
Thinking about the work group: nurses talk about themselves

The possibility of learning more about the often extremely painful, conflicting, and contradictory experiences within the work group is what carries the group's thought-process through the various phases described above and leads to the further development of the work. Through the mirror resonance process, the group attains the realization that "everyone's experience is different, and what appears externally does not always correspond to the real internal problem".

Nurses become aware that their behaviour and emotions do not only relate to children's situations and parents' experiences, but are also conditioned by their own personal problems. Hence the need to come up with their own real feelings during the meetings and to assess their nature even when they are destructive or aggressive. This is made possible by the fact that they feel supported by a competent work group, which is seen as the unbiased department–parent that opens its arms to everybody, the life-sustenance machine that provides enough hope and strength to maintain cohesiveness and to get on with the work.

On the one hand, awareness of the group's aggressive aspects is a positive feature, because it enables the group to attain a better integration of undesirable feelings and to make use of them. In consequence, the risk of acting out defence mechanisms, such as idealization and projection, is reduced. But, on the other hand, nurses express their clear concern about the cohesion of the group itself, which might be undermined by the expression of too violent or aggressive aspects.

> *Example:*   This meeting continues and develops the concerns of the previous one. Four nurses—Maria Gratia, Bambina, Lucia, and Anna—are present, together with a medical student and a student infant-neuropsychiatrist.
>
> Bambina says: "I would like to ask whether during today's meeting we could talk a bit about the problem of shyness."
>
> I say, "Yes, of course."
>
> Anna: "Everything started with an article we read in the newspaper, but which has little to do with shyness: it was the news about a robbery in a village near Treviglio, which resulted in the deaths of two people; one of them has just died in this hospital. I don't know how the problem emerged, but we have been wondering what shyness actually is."
>
> I answer: "It depends. . . ."

The nurses want to talk about themselves. A death has been caused by an act of aggression, and they want to know in what way aggressiveness operates as a defence against anxiety about death. They wonder: where do the attacks against the group, or within the group, go? What is the role played by destructiveness within the group? Is it possible to express it, can it be tolerated? Or will the group act in retaliation instead?

> Anna wonders: "What happens if someone becomes aggressive? Is it good or dangerous? What is shyness? If a person acts aggressively, is it a sign of self-assertiveness or of shyness?"

> Different nurses comment on this subject. Lucia regards aggressiveness as dangerous and presents a defence mechanism: "In my opinion, we're all the same; we are all shy—some more, some less." My intervention at this point is aimed at stopping them feeling directly responsible for it: "Many attitudes are conditioned by social factors. . . ."

> Then Lucia feels free to ask: "Can there be aggressive people or not?" And she implicitly asks: "What might happen?"

> I bring the problem back to internal aspects, while Maria Gratia clarifies that the problem of what might happen concerns the group: "There is a colleague of ours who is always so self-confident, so aggressive. . . ." It is as though she wanted to say: "We have got an effective group, and we are afraid that something might destroy it."

As already seen at the beginning of the session, the nurses believe that in their group, aggression is a negative element, which causes death; and they talk about the different ways in which they defend themselves from destructiveness. Destructiveness is the result of anxieties that could be related to the death instinct; shyness is an expression of internal conflicts, a manifestation of fear.

Analysing these problems, Bambina suggests "paralysis" and inhibition as a means of defence: "We are shy", she says, "because we do not know how to react when faced with a new situation." "It is true", adds Anna: "the feeling of shyness is basically fear." Lucia describes a defensive attitude, as before, which is not yet shared by her colleagues: "We all feel that way, we are all the same", she says. "Even doctors, when they first come to the department, feel insecure. . . . It seems to me such a universal feeling." She makes the very important distinction between "what can be seen outside—namely, action—and what is inside—namely, thought. . . . External appearances are not enough to tell whether someone is shy or not. They can just be masks."

At this point nurses start talking about their own experiences. They have been confronted with death, which is also inside us. They can go on, leaving the past behind for the unknown, for something new and important. But a certain fear creeps in that projections could undermine this new experience. "For example, at the beginning I felt uneasy. I had an internal crisis, which I also allowed to show, so making other people feel uneasy as well." Then Lucia and Bambina talk about their destructive feelings: but it is important to distinguish—as the student neuropsychiatrist pointed out—between "acting" and "the phantasy of acting".

It is also important to distinguish between "speaking" as an attempt to discharge tension and "speaking" as a means of communication and understanding. Through some examples brought by Lucia, we also saw how the anxiety brought about by fear of death heightens the risk of acting out aggressiveness; and how the nurses want their aggressiveness to be forgiven, because "when there is anxiety there is aggressiveness; otherwise there would be shyness".

We can see here how the setting-up of an effective group helps the nurses to preserve their internal objects, thus enabling them to talk about their own aggressiveness. Nevertheless, their fear of the consequences of their destructiveness and their concern to maintain the group's cohesion is always present.

Final conclusions

As time goes on, owing to the emotionally dramatic nature of the environment, the work group periodically re-experiences the thinking process that has been described in its various phases in this chapter. Again they will tackle the chaotic and persecutory aspects of the emotional atmosphere that prevent them from looking at the child as a whole. And again, ultimately, after working through that experience and the next phase concerning the neutral role, they will rediscover their ability to observe the child as an integrated being with biological and emotional components, and so they will be able to perform their caring function.

Given this approach, my own role in the group requires me to leave as much space as possible for the group members' contributions. Nevertheless, I take care to intervene when anxiety reaches high levels; and I also perform the secondary function of helping the group to distinguish, observe, associate and remember. (I am not supposed to interpret the psychodynamics of the group because it is not a therapy group, but I find it useful to adopt a psychoanalytic approach in observing and evaluating what is going on.)

The primary aim of the work is to help the staff to improve its threshold of tolerance to mental pain by recognizing and acknowledging it. To this end, I availed myself of my particular experience of infant observation, finding a space and role of my own within the group to accomplish my task—which was to promote the observation of very small children in distress; to enable nurses to direct their emotionality; to facilitate bonding; and, finally, to help them to live their relationship with the newborn fully. In turn, my own knowledge of child and parents is improved by listening to the nurses' comments. There is a mutual exchange of information which proves very stimulating and which radically changes the manner of caring for the infant. Also, as one's knowledge deepens, the urge to work thoroughly and to transform work into research becomes stronger.

The group takes part in this research and benefits from it through representing and understanding its own anxiety and becoming better able to observe the children in order to carry out more effectively the functions aimed at their recovery.

CHAPTER THREE

Infant observation

The observation of preterm newborns in the incubator from the first moments of their hospitalization was started in 1982. It was intended primarily as research for a medical university degree thesis, and also to improve the care of these infants. When starting this observation work, I believed that the recognition of extremely early mental mechanisms would provide a better understanding of the baby's distress and needs (Benedetti, 1984). It would enable more appropriate provision to be made of the various "direct preventive actions" I have identified, to improve its mental and physical condition during and after its stay in the incubator (as illustrated in Table 2, page 5).

Yet the initial approach to the early mental processes of a newborn who was so seriously premature and in such great distress soon brought into contact obscure aspects of the observer's mentality and more generally of all the people involved with the child. Our thoughts often tended to be fragmented and abortive. We felt strongly and painfully that parts of ourselves found it difficult to be psychologically born and to find their identity.

The observation work, therefore, starts in a difficult and tortuous way, then follows an unpredictable and uncharted route, which entails substantial changes in the practice of infant care, going far beyond what had originally been expected. In addition to what have been defined as "preventive environmental actions" on behalf of the child (Box 5), the observation work entailed a change in the mental approach of the staff regarding how to think about the child, and a deeper awareness and involvement on the part of the parents. As a result, the setting of the weekly meetings, the meeting procedures with parents, and my own neuropsychological evaluation of the child came to change substantially.

To understand the nature of this change and its consequences in the department, it is necessary to go back over the phases through which infant observation itself has evolved.

Methodological aspects

From a methodological point of view, the frequency of observation during the infant's early life corresponds with (but also differs from) that suggested by Esther Bick (1964). I noted that a single weekly observation for an ill newborn child does not allow one to follow its rapid changes and therefore the successive phases characterizing its development. So hour-long observations every other day were established throughout the child's hospitalization. Following the child's discharge from hospital, one weekly observation in the family was arranged, according to Esther Bick's prescribed method (Bick, 1964; Houzel, 1989; Lussana, 1984; Magagna, 1987; Negri, 1973, 1989a, 1989b; Perez Sanchez, 1990; Sandri, 1991). Performing the observation in the family (as she suggests) is not a casual choice; and in the case of the distressed preterm infant it corresponds to the neonatal intensive care unit, which is the natural environment for a child in that condition—the only place where it could survive at that point in its life. Here, infant observation would be devoid of all meaning if the nurses' care as well as the emotive presence of the parents (albeit not very

BOX 5

Preventive environmental actions

Unfortunately, preventive actions on behalf of the preterm newborn have up to now been based on the theory that it is deficient in sensory experience. The hyperstimulation to which it is subjected inside the incubator has never been sufficiently taken into account. In particular, according to Korner (1989), it is exposed to an excessively strong light and to monotonous noises. The medical intensive care procedures disrupt its sleep rhythm and at the same time provoke an oxygen desaturation. These factors must lead us to reflect on the importance and mode of stimulating actions—to what purpose, in what way, and at what intervals they should be carried out. For preventive environmental actions to be effective (see Table 2, page 5), they must take into account the newborn's gestational age, and appropriate actions must be applied in the best way. Gottlieb (1971), in studying the ontogenesis of the sense functions of birds and mammals, including man, has noted how the sensory system develops according to a specific constant developmental sequence, beginning with skin sensitivity in the oral or snout region and progressing to vestibular, acoustic, and visual functioning. Smell and taste start after the vestibular function, but before the hearing function (Gottlieb, 1971).

Sensory systems start working before the nervous structures are completely mature (Gottlieb, 1976; McGraw, 1946). This exerts a beneficial influence on the development of neural structures. Given that intrauterine life offers the most adequate stimulation for the ideal development of the foetus until the end of pregnancy, it is clear that those who care for the premature newborn (for whom these ideal conditions have abruptly come to an end) must consider what sensory functions have been interrupted. This will depend on the infant's gestational age, and preventive actions must be geared towards this, with the aim not of speeding up the child's development, but of maintaining and supporting it.

BOX 5

Preventive environmental actions (continued)

Initially the most necessary form of support is one that facilitates the organization of the child's states. Once this is accomplished, a more balanced relation with external modes of intervention becomes possible.

Our preventive environmental actions (see Table 2, page 5) produce both short- and long-term effects on the child's development. Both must be taken carefully into account. Short-term effects include changes in the child's clinical course, in its physiological functions, in the sleep–waking cycle, and in interactive behaviour. It is important to monitor the quality of the response to our intervention by checking the parameters indicating its well-being (heart-beat, respiratory activity, PO_2, and PCO_2). Long-terms results will be evaluated in collaboration with neonatologists during the follow-up, which lasts from the child's discharge from hospital until school age (Bondonio, 1981; Di Cagno et al., 1988; Ferrari, Sturloni, & Cavazzuti, 1984; Pisaturo & Ciravegna, 1983; Regini & Scavo, 1990).

---

active initially) were not taken into consideration. For this reason, parents and nurses are kept up to date about my work programme, and their spontaneous reactions are noted down as part of its progression. In turn, the observation material becomes an object of discussion during the weekly meetings that take place with the medical and non-medical staff of the department.

Difficulties of infant observation in the incubator

Several authors, including Esther Bick (1964) herself, but also Martha Harris (cited in Negri, 1973) and more recently Margaret Rustin (1988), have described the difficulties encountered in observing a healthy child in the context of its family.

These concern the child's emotions, which are so intense during its first period of development that they interfere with the observer's perceptive capacity, thus altering the quality of the observation itself. Such difficulties become even more pressing in the environment of the neonatal intensive care unit, where the newborn often finds itself in a painful and extremely critical condition, struggling to survive. It is not easy to observe a motionless child undergoing invasive and bloody therapeutic procedures. As a mother once expressed it in an interview, the child conjures up the image of a fragile little monkey undergoing vivisection. But for a seriously premature newborn, that is not all. As the literature often stresses (Garcia Coll, 1990; Gorski, Huntington, & Lewkowicz, 1990; Lester et al., 1990; Tronick et al., 1990), as well as appearing a fragile and suffering creature, for a long time the child will show a peculiar inadequacy in its ability to react and interact. It can pass from an absolute inability to respond to even nociceptive stimuli generated by its environment (hypo-reactivity) to an excessive response to specific actions (hyper-reactivity).

By comparison with the child born at term, the preterm newborn is in the early period much less alert, reactive, and socially responsive. What is specially highlighted in the literature is its extremely poor ability to interact with those who take care of it. Thus it is soon evident how difficult it is to observe a creature at this stage of development. It is a painful experience to tolerate, because one is confronted with embryonic features of mental activity.

This experience is shared by all those who surround the newborn—observer, doctors, nurses, and parents alike. Anxieties about death and the possibility that life may indeed not prevail have a paralysing effect and interfere with one seeing the child as a living creature; consequently, one feels unable to help it survive. One feels powerless when confronted with this struggle. The child is truly struggling for survival, therefore one identifies with it and feels a sense of rebellion.

Generally in our perception of relationships we help each other, using as a medium some aspect of the other person, like a placenta that allows us to establish a contact through which to deepen our knowledge. But the preterm newborn, during its first period of life, offers the observer nothing directly lively to cling on to; it is difficult to detect any vital elements or find any response. Looking at the creature lying in the incubator, it seems impossible to think and maintain a "fluctuating" attention level. So, during this first observation phase, one is baffled by a violent and intense frustration, which is difficult to tolerate.

Inevitably, there is a temptation to engage in mechanisms of defence. The observer may find himself producing an accurate and detailed description from a distance, identifying isolated functions but failing to grasp the nature of the object of observation itself—namely, the child. We can see this in the following observation made by a medical student of a baby girl born at 30 weeks, weighing 1.170 kg:

> "The girl makes a segmentary movement with her right foot only, which she bends and extends a couple of times; then she stops the right foot and repeats the same movement with her left foot, and then again with her right one. She bends her right leg, bringing it towards her thigh. She moves her mouth as though she were sucking. She tries to take off her little glove from her left hand, by means of abduction and adduction movements of her elbow towards her trunk. Then she extends her left arm until she touches the incubator wall with her left hand."

The frequent use of terms borrowed from medical jargon (abduction, adduction, segmentary movements) does not help us to detect even prognostically meaningful data about the functioning ability of the nervous system.

Milani Comparetti (1982a, 1982b) defines as motor development only the acquisition of primary automatisms, the outcome of an epigenetic mechanism. Primary automatisms, being genetically programmed functions, are the predetermined responses of the species to fundamentally psychic problems evoked by the environment. The static repertoire of primary automatisms remains the same for all individuals belonging to the same species, whereas observation of motor development in the foetus now indicates to us that the foetus is reacting to its environment with the uniqueness of an individual. It shows a primary motivated competence in action, which is quite distinct from anything in the reflexological and behavioural models of the mind at this stage. The constant factor in the ontogenetic process and in motor development seems to be the structural role played by the individual, who projects himself towards the surrounding world and creates himself with his "propositional competence" (Box 6).

Examination of the child must, therefore, be founded on a search for "propositional competence" and not on its ability to make purposeless movements or to respond to stimuli. It is not

---

BOX 6

Milani Comparetti's "propositional competence"

Milani Comparetti (1982a, 1982b) states that observation of the foetus's motor development suggests that the individual predominates over the environment, thus stressing the individual's primary competence in action. This view is in opposition to the environment-dependent reflexological and behavioural models. A constant feature of the ontogenetic process and of motor behaviour seems to be the essential role of the living being projecting itself onto the surrounding world and creating itself by means of its propositional competence. Emde (1988) identifies similar attributes in the young child, which can be summed up under three categories: (1) the "activity", which refers to how sensori-motor activities express intrinsic purposes—the first most fundamental evidence of motivation; (2) "self-regulation", which in the short term (in addition to the vital systems such as the cardiorespiratory and metabolic) regulates attention, wakefulness, and the sleep–waking cycles, and in the long term regulates the functions of growth and development; (3) "social fitness", which describes the intrinsic organizational ability of our species in establishing, maintaining, and fulfilling interaction with other individuals.

In 1985, Stern described a concept similar to the "propositional competence" [*competenza propositiva*] of Milani Comparetti (1982a, 1982b), in the context of the 2- to 6-month-old child. He stated that in order to attain its "nuclear self", the child must possess an "acting self".

at all easy to conduct a child observation from the right mental distance: finding a position that is not stable and definitive, but is sufficiently detached to metabolize what had previously been obstacles, so that these can improve the quality of our knowledge-seeking instruments.

The first period

During its first days of life, the newborn appears to suffer a great deal, owing to its pathological condition of serious prematurity and to all the medical interference it must undergo in order to survive. (The definition of a seriously preterm newborn applies to a child born before the 32nd week of gestation. At present, even infants born at the 25th week of gestation can succeed in surviving. Their weight is lower than 1000 g, and they are defined as ELBWI (Extremely Low Birth Weight Infants) by American authors.) Here is the first observation of Giacomo, a baby born at 25 weeks and 3 days, weighing 780 g. I saw him for the first time two days after his birth.

The observation was intense and energy-consuming; the newborn's suffering was clearly evident:

> *Giacomo:* "He is a minute, fragile, very delicate child, with a suffering and emaciated look. He has a very thin face, with regular features. His face is immobile, but in spite of that, it gives the impression of great suffering. He is in a supine position, with his arms and legs stretched inside the incubator. His abdomen shows clear signs of abrasion on the skin. He is immobile. Only from time to time can very slight movements of his left foot be observed."

The difficulty I experienced in observing this child was in keeping my attention focused on him, while at the same time feeling overwhelmed by anxiety for the child. But I realize that I will only be able to communicate with him if I manage to combine the emotional experience simultaneously with the sense experience of continuing to look at him.

The child's distress, and his immobility—due to the fact that each individual gesture would cost him too much energy—might lead one to believe that he is not alive, even though he is alive. In these circumstances the important thing is to learn to perceive the slightest changes, such as those from the state of utter immobility to the moment of moving his little foot. The main means of expression of these tiny children is their motility. It is interesting to imagine the connection between their inner life and their type of motility; but at this level it is difficult for those taking care of the child not to consider its body as a machine; for the intolerable anxiety aroused by the critical condition of the child can cause a split in one's perception, separating its body from its mental activity.

There are very few means of trying to make the child's stay in the incubator more tolerable at this very early stage. The following procedures, mentioned earlier, can help: the use of a lamb's fleece to lie on (Scott et al., 1983; Scott & Martin, 1981), a little sheet to protect the child from the ambient light, taste stimulation, and sound therapy to break the monotony and deflect the disturbing noise inside the incubator (Box 7) (Bess, Peek, & Chapman, 1979; Peltzam et al., 1970). We try to place

---

BOX 7

Sound therapy

From the very beginning, a tape with the recording of the maternal heart-beat, as the baby has it *in utero*, is placed in the incubator (Salk, 1973). In addition, parents are asked to record a tape with anything they might wish on it: music, verbal messages, etc. The tape is then introduced inside the incubator, so the child can listen to it (De Casper & Fifer, 1980).

The significance of this intervention for the parents is discussed in chapter one. As far as the child is concerned, the aim of the tape is to sooth it and let it feel that the parents are close to it.

the baby in its favourite positions, if the equipment to which he is connected allows it. Too much interference would incur the risk of overloading it with stimuli, given the continuous presence of all the equipment necessary for its survival.

The child's suffering

The child's suffering, especially during the first days of its admission, emerges very clearly in the following observation of Giacomo.

> Giacomo is now the equivalent of 26 weeks and 4 days. He is always immobile, supine, with legs and arms spread out. A hiccup shakes him, and his face shows frequent grimaces. He is very irritated by the bronchial suctioning manoeuvres; he reacts by kicking, when an electrode is removed from his abdomen. I feel almost paralysed by anxiety at the sight of such a distressed baby. I realize how difficult it is to conduct the observation.

> I feel painfully constrained by a clash with primitive and obscure mental processes of my own. In the presence of this defenceless creature's suffering, my own mental equipment and the instruments available to me as a person responsible for undertaking reparative action seem hopelessly limited. I often turn my eyes away from the child to scrutinize the equipment displaying his state of health. Today, for the first time in three observations, I note three big warts near his left ear. But what strikes me most is the sense that time stands still during the moments when I am actually looking at Giacomo.

> From this session onwards, my presence motivates the nurse to come close to the incubator repeatedly and for longer, whereas before I noticed that she would approach the baby only if the machines detected a problem. While I am concentrating on the child's suffering, trying to be absorbed by it, the nurse comments on his signs of malaise as though they referred automatically to his physical state: the shaking diaphragm is

due to the catarrh that obstructs the tube and therefore secre-
tions need to be aspirated, etc. My presence, respecting the
child's suffering, and the nurse's attention to the child's bodily
expressions constitute the first simultaneous approach to the
child's body and mind together. But as yet these two aspects
are not integrated within the nurse's perception; the suffering
still prevents the nurse from seeing the child, confining her to
descriptions of the child's vital functions—breathing, heart
beat, etc. Yet her comment about his good adjustment to the
respirator, which became noticeable from the end of the session, also includes another meaning, if we consider the psychopathological risks. For it is very important that the child should
adapt to the respirator, as this will lead to an improved sense of
well-being. If he is opposed to it, his suffering, restlessness,
distress, and irritability will increase.

The child's physiognomy

The "propositional competence" of the preterm newborn; the projection and the attachment of significance by nurses

As time passes and the physical condition of the preterm newborn improves, towards the 29th–30th week of gestational age,
observation of the child allows me to recognize some of the
features that will characterize it in the future. These initial
expressions of vitality have immediate repercussions in terms
of the more complex and active mental functioning of those who
surround the child. Through the child's recovery the nurses
also recover the normal and natural projective functions of
communication and of the attachment of significance. In fact,
the mental functions of the nursing staff record the extent of
the child's vitality rather like an X-ray photograph. This X-ray
metaphor also illustrates the parallel I observed in myself
between the improvement in the child's vital functions and the
change in my own mentality as observer. The nurses themselves seem to be well aware of this. One nurse, who was about
to administer one of three daily intramuscular injections to a

preterm girl weighing 820 g, commented that she hoped Marta's lungs would improve, so the child would feel better and in consequence so would she, because she would no longer have to inject her.

I believe that initially at this early stage the nurses are inclined to think of the life of the newborn in an automatic and mechanical way, not just because of the intolerable anxiety aroused by the child, but also because they are well aware of the suffering they themselves inflict through their therapeutic manipulations. Those taking care of the child need to protect their own minds from too massive an identification with the little patient. This could seriously impair their ability to carry out their work. On the other hand, being able to actively improve the child's well-being is a real source of relief for the nurses.

At this stage my own situation as observer is different, because I cannot take active measures to improve the child's health, so am confined solely to having to think about what is happening to the child. Nevertheless, comments made by nurses during the observation, and the transformation of the treatment work afterwards, show how my presence near the incubator—the fact of being "with" the child—conveyed a sense of safety about their ability to formulate thoughts concerning the child. It is as though the fact that there is someone who thinks about the patient and holds it in mind makes it possible for all those around it to think about the child too. If someone can think about what is happening to the child, everyone can do it: a sort of circle of thought takes shape, enwrapping the child and involving all the people present: observer, doctors, nurses, and parents. So if what Dr Corominas (1983b) has stated is true—that if a child is thought about, it will develop— then the premature newborn will benefit from this. (This also has very important implications for a problem related to the treatment of terminally ill patients, which cannot be dealt with here, but which has made a remarkable contribution to treatment in the neonatal pathology division where I work.)

The first signs of any interest in the "outside" on the part of the child are very significant in its development, because then one can try to offer a comprehensible response to these primitive means of communication, and to ease its condition through the preventive environmental actions already mentioned (Minde et al., 1978). Some children, such as Giacomo, like eye-contact; others prefer to use other senses for their interaction with the environment, such as hearing, sucking, or grasping with hands or feet, or skin sensations—the pleasure of being caressed and handled. Thus Giacomo, from the session when he was 28 weeks and 6 days (gestational age), began to keep his eyes wide open and turned outwards more often and for a longer time. The nurses made lively, affectionate, and imaginative comments on this, saying: "From the very beginning, Giacomo's eyes followed everything; the day he was reintubated, he was looking at us to see what we were doing. We were petrified while looking at him—it seemed as though he were checking on us; usually children are so upset by reintubation that they keep their eyes closed. It is really incredible, he is so sensitive and loves being fondled; but what has struck us most from the first day is his eyes—he is so curious to see everything" (Box 8).

So from this session of 28 weeks 6 days onwards, when the death risk has been reduced, we find ourselves in a different situation with Giacomo during observations. Now during the observation he often has his big dark eyes wide open, and they seem to look "above" or "up towards us". A slight increase in vitality in the child results in a change in the mental state of the group, so it resumes its function of thinking about the child as a living being equipped with specific sensorial attributes and with his own "propositional competences". In consequence, the nurses make comments that show that they consider Giacomo as a proper individual child, eager for experience and interested in the outside world: "He does not like being manipulated." The nurses also point out his need for freedom, when they say: "He fights the respirator, the tube hinders him; he seems relieved when you take it off."

During this stage of observation, attention to the equipment connected to the newborn lessens in priority, and the child starts directing embryonic messages towards its environment. The observer perceives a differentiating mental activity in these, and the nurses start to attribute meanings to the child's

BOX 8

The mother's presence near the incubator
(observations of Minde, Tronick, and myself)

From the first day of his hospitalization, Giacomo was lucky to have the presence of his mother and often his father near the incubator. His parents' presence proved a positive stimulation for his interaction with the outside environment. Minde (Minde et al., 1978) observed that the newborns who keep their eyes open most are those who are cuddled and touched most often by their mothers.

My own observation experience of seriously premature newborns does not allow me to agree with Minde fully. I agree that those newborns whose parents are not often in attendance near the incubator tend to express interest more in the inside of the incubator than in the outside. But I have also observed infants with analogous gestational age and pathology who—though their mothers may likewise be often near them—spend most of their time inside the incubator asleep, and they have waking periods of only a very few moments. We might note here that sleeping can be a defence against unsatisfactory living conditions. These are children who can benefit from environment-generated sensory stimulation such as caressing and the water mattress, but who use it in order to fall asleep more easily. This observation is confirmed by the research work done by Tronick et al. (1990), when they refer to a condition of "protective apathy". This can be seen in some preterm newborns as a means of conserving useful energy in order to achieve and maintain homeostasis and so aid recovery.

slight movements. The ambience is enriched with meaningfulness; the nurses seem to anticipate the child's "propositional competence", which will appear clearly to the observer from the 32nd week (of gestational age).

As the child develops its "propositional competence" in connection with the integration and organization of sensorial

functions, it is noticeable that the people around start respond-
ing with everyday reflections: linking the degree of the child's
competence with common sense. In "common sense" a tradi-
tion of experience needs to be discovered and lived out. At this
stage it would be an exaggeration to talk about the child's
"intentionality", but we are moving in this direction in considering the specificity of the child's initiative, enriched with
significance. From an epistemological point of view we need a
way of defining qualitatively the first manifestations of something that later becomes expressed in a more organized way
through intention and will. If we make use of "common sense",
we can imagine that the child is already at this stage equipped
with "propositional competence". We need to grasp this sudden
feeling, despite the poor organization of its behaviour, of the
child's move towards a more integrated and meaningful mode
of experience.

The image of the living child
in the parents' mind

For those parents who are able to follow their child's long
experience in the incubator closely, even the slightest increase
in vitality, the slightest outward movements, help them to
contain and overcome their anxiety for their endangered child
and to build up an image of a live and beautiful child. This
experience is very important for the parent–child relationship,
since it allows the realization of what Meltzer (Meltzer & Harris
Williams, 1988) has defined as the "aesthetic conflict" to take
place, which is essential for the child's emotional development.
It is difficult for this experience to take place with such a frail,
distressed, and barely vital creature as the preterm newborn.

> During this observation session, when Giacomo is 30
> weeks of gestational age, both parents are near the
> incubator. They are visibly moved: the father shows great
> interest and knowledgeability about the machines that
> keep his child alive and talks with the nurses about them.
> The mother concentrates more on her child. But they are

both interested in my observation of Giacomo. Today he weighs 1260 g. He immediately opens his eyes and for a moment seems to look up at us while we observe him, then shakes his limbs slightly, sticks out his tongue, makes a gentle movement, and acts as if he wanted to "get up". His mother expresses her strong desire to take him out of the incubator and lift him in her arms. Then he starts sleeping quietly again. His father says: "I feel a glimmer of hope about his life starting . . . last autumn I came here to this hospital for two months, taking care of my dying father. That is why I named my son Giacomo." The child gives a start; his father places his hand in the incubator and strokes his nose. After a while he opens his eyes again and seems to look up at his father, who says meanwhile: "What a beautiful child he is. . . . I can't remember when he was tiny. . . ."

When the child raises his eyes, it is noticeable how the parents' anxiety for its survival lessens; this is a child that can be talked to and seen as beautiful. The parents find him beautiful, which means that the tension deriving from anxieties about death has been overcome. Now they dare observe his physique: it is better; he is now able to "look"; and if *he* looks, then the father in response can start to notice his child's qualities. We can see that the same evolution of thought that had occurred in the observer and the nurses is now taking place in the parents. The minds of all of them are no longer riddled by fear of death. Not only does the equipment give hopeful data about the child, but also the descriptions coming from the human mental environment confirm this.

I can trace the change in my thought orientation as observer by reading my accounts of the sessions. From now on the descriptions become more fluid and dynamic, in response to the child's "propositional competence" and evidence of growth and development. They are quite different from the description of the first sessions, where the child's initial actions often appear to be fragmented. From a prognostic point of view, it is very significant when parents come up with memories, such as when Giacomo's father talks about his father's death as an event in the past—clearly showing that the anxiety about death has been allayed.

The child's states of irritability and first mental movements: object differentiation

In the period between the 30th and 32nd weeks, some irritation and moments of restlessness can be seen in the child. His age and improved clinical condition give him greater vitality, and he finds it difficult to tolerate the assisted respiration (Box 9) and is annoyed by the tubes of the ventilator and the feeding tube. However, he is not always able to breathe without the aid of the mechanical equipment, so he cannot do without it.

Even at this stage it is not easy to help the child overcome these irritating moments. We always try to find the most suitable posture for him, provide him with the sheep's fleece, non-nutritional sucking, caresses, and sound therapy (see Box 7, p. 89). Naturally the procedures that the child seems to prefer and find most relieving are applied. However, observations made at this time indicate not only physical restlessness but also the first embryonic signs of a need for "the other"—for interaction and relationship. To illustrate this, I will quote from Giacomo's 31-week session:

> He is lying supine on the lamb's fleece; he is still intubated and still has the feeding tube, and he is wearing his little gloves. He weighs 1260 g. The nurse near the incubator tells me: "He is still restless. He has been listening to the music tape-recorded by his mother for four days, but it is hard to know whether he likes it or not. He is very lively, but he does not want to breathe. He is fat! He had a blood

---

BOX 9

Artificial ventilation

This is a necessary procedure to ensure the respiratory functioning of seriously preterm newborns affected by lung immaturity, or of infants born at term affected by a serious lung disorder (aspiration syndrome, bronchopneumonia, pneumothorax) or a serious neurological disability.

transfusion test yesterday. Also he has a healthy complexion. He is asleep but will soon wake up; he can't sleep for a very long time."

In fact, today Giacomo is sleeping very lightly. Now he has his eyes wide open, moves them, and seems to be looking around. He sleeps without moving, very quietly, to the sound of "music relaxation". His mouth opens, he draws his legs up towards his tummy, slightly moves his arms, then becomes motionless again. His breath is irregular, but a nurse tells me: "His fight against the respirator does not last long; if left to himself, Giacomo soon gives up. . . ."

This session helps us to understand what an increase in vitality means for the baby at this stage of development. It seems it is not just a question of movement, of being able to look. If we consider the implications of the nurse's comment that if left to himself Giacomo soon "gives up", we realize that the child's vitality seems inextricable from a request for somebody to act. Vitality, therefore, is more than just movement, automatism, respiration in themselves; it also includes an outward tension, a need to establish a relation with someone. So we see in the case of Giacomo two contrasting conceptions of vitality: one that involves reacting with someone else, and the other consisting in his needing to do everything alone and deciding to throw the respirator away.

Later on, he stretches himself, and the nurse comments: "He is wet; that's why he is annoyed and starts getting up." Indeed, he is moving his bottom and becoming very restless. "He's always done this, even before, when he wasn't really strong enough." The little sheet is gently changed. He becomes quiet again. The nurse speaks of trying to wean him from the respirator: "He has been trying for a week, but he has never managed it. Carla, on the other hand, showed more determination." (Carla, a seriously preterm child born at 26 weeks and 5 days, weighing 920 g, left the department ten days before Giacomo's arrival. Already at 29 weeks she was able to breathe alone and achieved a rapid adjustment to the day-

and-night cycle through an early satisfactory organization of biological rhythms.)

Giacomo, therefore, tries to get away from what most bothers him immediately—wee and poo—whereas he tolerates his reliance on the respirator on which his survival has depended. He starts to throw away everything he can, as though he already had an early perception of the disturbing, bad object, but will not release the object he depends on. So the good object/respirator correlation and the bad object/sheet with wee and poo correlation start to take shape. Giacomo's dependence worries the nurses because if it becomes excessive, it can turn into a lung complication; it seems that the baby has not intuited this risk yet.

Removal of the tracheal tube: a second birth

The early processes of introjection

Extubation is a crucial moment during the newborn's period in hospital and is usually pursued with deep involvement by the medical and non-medical staff and by the parents. On the one hand it is clear that artificial ventilation is necessary for the child's survival; on the other hand, it can in the long term become a serious obstacle. Parents usually look forward to the tube being removed, but when the time comes closer they are filled with panic and anxiety. They are afraid that their child will not manage to breathe alone and that he might die. In this period it is advisable to increase the interviews with parents, and it is not unusual for them to bring frightening dreams.

The nurses' state of mind is different, because they are well aware of the risks the child would incur if he depended on the respirator for too long. The thinking focused on the child in the context of this event is very warm and loving. A substantial change is about to take place in the child's life and in the way the nurses and parents will look on him. "Once you have removed it", said one nurse referring to the respirator, "it is as though he were born again." The event is tantamount to a new birth. We can illustrate this through the observation of Giacomo:

> During the session at 31 weeks and 4 days, Giacomo is extubated. Only the little continuous pressure tube remains, together with the feeding tube. Today he weighs 1.270 kg. His mother, who is very anxious, is near the incubator. She tells me that Giacomo has been restless all day long, and shows me the c.p.p. tube as being the cause of the problem (Box 10). She fears that the baby will not make it, will not be able to breathe alone. The nurse who is with us says, as if in answer to Giacomo's mother, that during the next few days, while the change in respiration is being established, Giacomo must be stimulated—he cannot sleep too much. Indeed, he cannot lie on his tummy—his favourite position—because of the c.p.p. tube, and that is why he is so irritable (Box 11).

This is a very special observation session: three of us are around the incubator—myself as silent observer; the mother who is visibly anxious; and the nurse, who is explaining the meaning of what the child is doing at this critical point in his

---

BOX 10

Continuous positive pressure endonasal tube

This is a support procedure (in non-seriously preterm newborns or in newborns born at term) in minor respiration impairments or in pathological patterns characterized by relapsing apnoeas. It is also applied in the phase following extubation of the infant who had required artificial ventilation. This procedure involves the inflation of air-oxygen to dilate the pulmonary alveoli and, more generally, to promote spontaneous breathing. It is an irritating procedure for the infant owing to constriction of the tube, possible lesions of the nasal mucosae, and possible stomach dilation, with feeding troubles.

BOX 11
The water mattress

After extubation, Giacomo showed constant restlessness when the continuous pressure tube was applied to him. The water mattress was used at this point, with the satisfactory results seen over the past six years: when the preterm newborn is laid on the water mattress, which tends to fluctuate according to the baby's own movements, it attains a condition of calm and well-being more easily.

Korner and colleagues (1975, 1978, 1983, 1989) have made particular studies of the advantages to be derived from vestibular and proprioceptive afferent impulses delivered to the newborn. These types of stimulation not only accelerate clinical recovery (in particular of the respiratory function), but, according to the author, they also encourage a better integration of sensori-motor functions, thus facilitating the child's development. My personal findings corroborate this observation. I personally assessed the benefit of submitting the premature newborn to vestibular stimulation through head-to-foot oscillation, induced by rhythmical pressure on the water mattress where the child was lying. This procedure seems to be advantageous not only in reducing the number of apnoeas, but also in providing the child with stimuli analogous to those received by the foetus in intrauterine life.

life. My silent presence and the nurses' comments seem to help the mother to overcome her initial anxiety, letting her give shape to phantasies about the baby when he was still inside her: "She imagined she heard her baby call her 'mummy', soon after the child's conception." The nurse explicitly stresses Giacomo's vitality, saying how he "likes sucking, likes being free to move, not constrained, likes having his nose stroked and leading a comfortable life". Only then, when there is a clear and optimistic picture of his chances of survival, does the mother start to look at the actual figure of the child and to recognize his vitality. She tells me that for 6 days he has begun to turn his eyes if someone called him through the porthole in the incubator, and for 15 days he has seemed to show interest in what is going on around him. Both nurse and mother carry on adding comments and observations, confirming the fact that the child really has made contact with the world.

The mother, therefore, shows she can distinguish the phantasies she had about her child inside her from her actual observations of the child. In those phantasies, Giacomo was seen as a part of herself, whereas her observations on her baby refer to the baby's own attributes. The differentiating function is clear.

Then, to return to the child itself during the session, we saw the primordial grasping function (also observed in other sessions); according to the nurse, this is because the child is nervous; he is disturbed by the little c.p.p. tube and by a noise to which he reacts with a start. The nurse perceives Giacomo's discomfort and says that at such times he has been soothed by sucking a piece of gauze soaked in glucose water (Box 12). Indeed, after this he is calmer and does not fidget, with his mouth open and his eyes half-open; then he grasps the little feeding tube with his hands. His foot makes a similar move-

---

BOX 12

Taste stimulation

Within the framework of what I define as preventive environmental actions (see Table 2, page 5) a fundamental role is played by taste stimulation—the sweetened water given to the child through a piece of gauze placed by its lips, and the rosehip syrup spread on the little finger of the mother or nurse, or on the teat of a tiny dummy belonging to a "Nati Ora" doll, which is used in our department owing to its minute size.

Taste shows itself to be a function that facilitates introjection and also helps in promoting the child's organization, since it is a great source of satisfaction for him. This sense of satisfaction, whenever possible, is an important feature of preventive action.

ment, touching the incubator wall. By grasping, he seems to be willing to relate himself to the object.

It is interesting to note that while the baby was grabbing at the little tube with his hands and seeking for contact with the wall by means of his foot, the nurse was completing our picture of a child who likes grasping things by adding her description of his enjoyment of sucking sweetened water. Sucking is one of the most common ways for the newborn to develop its intro-jective processes. In this way the nurse seemed to confirm my interpretation of the child's earliest introjective processes be-ginning to emerge (Box 13). It should be pointed out that Giacomo can only suck if the gauze is held to his mouth by the nurse, implying an early dependence experience. However, his mouth is not free to search for the object to suck, because for therapeutic purposes his head is still kept immobile.

The child's abrupt starting; grasping; the child's sleep

In the period between the 32nd and the 34th week of gesta-tional age, it is common to observe the newborn during long periods of sleep (Box 14). Sometimes a series of jerks interrupt the baby's sleep, and sometimes, as in the session described below, these can give its sleep a dramatic character.

At 32 weeks and 4 days, Giacomo weighs 1.350 kg. He seems much bigger and more beautiful. He is no longer completely naked, wearing a nappy around his waist. "He looks like a little schoolboy", the nurse says as she accompanies me to the incubator (Box 15).

Today the child has only the feeding tube. He is lying face down. It has been possible for him to keep this position for four days. He lies across the incubator, with his head against the wall. "He walks about in the incubator. He likes this position; he oxygenates better this way", the nurse remarks. She repositions him straight in the middle of the cot. He is still lying face down, with his mouth open.

BOX 13

Early processes of introjection and projection

Beginning at 28 weeks, Giacomo opens his eyes often and for
a long time. During the observation sessions at 31 weeks and
4 days, and the week after, I observed Giacomo's hands
grabbing the feeding tube and the sheet, and his foot touching the incubator wall. I interpreted these movements as the
earliest searching for an object. In the following sessions,
Giacomo made two new types of movement: sliding movements, through which he could explore the inside of the
incubator, and searching around for a way of supporting his
little foot. In the framework of the session, these two movements—of clinging and of looking for a support—seem to
anticipate introjection and projection.

These thoughts seem to be confirmed by ultrasonic observations that I have made on two pairs of non-identical twins.
These observations were continued after birth until the age of
2 years, following the method of Esther Bick. Both series of
observations, which have been supervised by Dr Meltzer,
gave us the opportunity, starting at 17 weeks of gestation, to
see a more definite expression of the same movements interpreted in Giacomo as marking an early process of introjection.

This occurred in the case of Elisa, the girl in the first pair of
twins, and Stefano, the boy in the second pair. In the ultrasound sessions we were struck by the way in which Elisa
related to the placenta and to her little brother as an object;
we were impressed by her intent eye movements, by her
grabbing with her hands and searching continuously for
sensuous contact with these two objects. This eye mobility
and the prehensile movements of hands and mouth at such
an early stage of development were so marked that they were
astonishing to behold. Similarly, Stefano, in the second pair
of twins, chose from 17 weeks on (unlike his sister Silvia) to
stay in one particular corner of the womb under the mother's

liver, in front of the placenta, in which he manifested a continuous interest: he often grabbed it, poked it, touched it with his hands, always keeping his face and head in close contact, throughout the sessions.

The other two twins, Daniele and Silvia, by contrast, showed no specific tendency to relate to an object, even though they showed a similar motor ability to the other twin in their pair.

Thus intent eye movements and a particular prehensile activeness in the mouth and hands could be observed in two of these foetuses, especially in Elisa. A frequent opening and closing of the mouth could also be observed in Giacomo: from the very beginning, he showed a special preference for sucking, when he was offered the piece of gauze with sweetened water.

It is worth remembering that the intrauterine life of the foetus is different from that of the life of a preterm newborn of similar gestational age. During the first days of the newborn's hospitalization, the search movements of his mouth are hampered; the child is forced to remain motionless to keep the ventilator tube in position.

The observation sessions carried out after the birth of the two pairs of twins, and of Giacomo later in his mother's arms and then at home after discharge, confirmed the particular inclination towards introjective processes that had emerged during intrauterine life with two of the twins, and which showed clearly in Giacomo from 30 weeks' gestational age.

The observation of the two pairs of twins and of several seriously preterm newborns leads us to assume that the specific inclination towards introjective and projective processes occurs in those babies who seem to have a good internal object from a very early stage in their foetal life. This leads to the assumption that the presence of an internal object for reference seems to be a hereditarily transmitted characteristic.

BOX 14

Ontogenesis of the sleep–waking cycles

Between the 24th and 27th weeks, no distinction can be made between sleeping and waking states. Dreyfus-Brisac (1970) has pointed out that, from 24 weeks on, a state of motion associated with crying can be observed, which could be regarded as the preliminary stage of the waking state.

Between the 29th and 30th weeks, an undifferentiated sleep can be observed. This is defined as transitional or indeterminate sleep. The main active behavioural characteristics of sleep can already be recognized, while the quiet sleep is hardly present at all. Between the 32nd and 36th week, the active sleep is well differentiated by REM, erratic respiration, and rough body movements; EEG displays a continuous activity. The quiet sleep emerges: it is characterized by a reduction in body motion, regular respiration, chin movements; EEG is discontinuous. Short periods of waking with a continuous EEG pattern can be seen; indeterminate sleep stages are fewer.

At 36 weeks, the waking state is well differentiated, and the active sleep–waking cycles and quiet stages of sleep can be clearly distinguished (Ferrari et al., 1984).

He sleeps leaning his head on his left cheek. He seems to smile frequently and intensely in his sleep (American authors refer to "reflex smiles"). He seems to smile and moves his hands. Then he moves his right hand under the sheet to grab the lamb's fleece beneath him. He jerks suddenly, making his left leg and right arm shiver. He is panting. Rhythmically he repeats the same grimace. He moves the toes of his right foot, then his legs and feet alternately. Then he becomes quiet again. He shakes his arms; he grabs the lamb's fleece with his left hand. He becomes motionless again.

Throughout this sequence, the baby reminds me of Esther Bick's description of a child being pursued by the threat of disintegration. How may such a tiny child be affected by such a process? He seems to be experiencing disturbing bodily sensations. What levels of suffering may exist in a nervous system not yet fully developed? What defences may such a small creature have? Giacomo seems to respond to what looks like the threat of disintegration by grabbing the lamb's fleece, the sheets of the cot. In this instance his grabbing action seems to be a primordial element, different from the grasping action of the hand that accompanies the movement of the mouth sucking the nipple—a later evolutionary stage, which for the newborn parallels the function of the mouth.

The primordial type of grasping occurs also with other parts of the newborn's body, such as the foot clinging onto the incubator. As already observed, the grabbing action that seems to be the first way of relating to the object seems to stem in this case from a painful experience. While I am observing this, the nurse does not notice the child's dramatic inquietude; she is still talking about him, as in the first part of the session, as like

---

BOX 15

The little schoolboy

The nurses' impression, almost always shared by parents, that the baby wearing a nappy "looks like a little schoolboy", was considered by the work group. The discussion pointed out the usefulness of preparing caps and socks made of coloured wool in which to dress the newborn from the beginning of his hospital admission. This is already done in several neonatal intensive care units, since it improves the overall thermoregulation of the newborn during the initial period. At the same time, we thought it might be experienced very positively by the parents. The first caps and socks were knitted by the nurses during their free time on night shifts and were placed on Marta, the preterm infant described in Box 22 (page 127).

a grown-up boy; and when Giacomo now wakes up, the nurse remarks: "He has a beautiful and lively look."

Again he is seized by sudden jerks, which make his lower limbs shiver; he then moves restlessly; first his legs and arms shake simultaneously, then they shiver separately.

At this point the nurse makes some remarks about the child's sleep: "He sleeps well since the tubes were removed." Now he just has little jerks of his left foot. His leg still shakes, then becomes quiet again.

The nurse does not perceive the suffering evidenced during the child's sleep. Not giving too much importance to this disturbance could be seen as a sign of confidence and hope. Yet I have the impression that this not-seeing reveals a sort of rejection of the idea of a mental life existing at this stage: a mind that is complex enough to be able to remember. It is as though the nurse unconsciously does not want the child to retain these painful memories.

The child's first waking moments; the nurses start to separate from the child

During the 32nd week, the child's first periods of wakefulness begin. In Giacomo's observation session at 32 weeks and 4 days (reported above), the nurse remarked that the child when he woke up was beautiful and lively. It is important at this stage to bear in mind the various states the child may be in: the prevailing active sleep alternates with periods of quiet sleep, and as in Giacomo's case, the first waking moments appear (Box 16). From the 32nd week, once physiological homeostasis has been reached, a regular pattern of phases of sleeping and waking begins to take place and the child appears increasingly more lively (Aylward, 1981).

The nurses soon take stock of these developments; they feel that he is now almost out of danger and therefore increasingly less dependent on their care. His mother is there, often both

BOX 16

Sleep–waking organization

From a prognostic point of view, once homeostasis has been achieved, the organization of the different states towards the 42nd week is a milestone for the development of the preterm child's mental health. The child's states can be defined as organized once he can remain in a well-defined state for significant periods, with a gradual shift from one to the other. Sudden changes of state signal the child's vulnerability, as can its motor and postural behaviour (Brazelton, 1973, 1984; Faienza, 1984; Faienza & Capone, 1993; Korner et al., 1988; Prechtl & Beintema, 1964; Wolff, 1966).

parents, and the staff realize how much strength the child has drawn from their presence.

During the session at 33 weeks and 2 days, they also connect his ability to pay attention to what is happening outside to his mother's presence, supporting him. In her turn, the mother has also felt encouraged by the nurses' and by my presence. They recognize that Giacomo is full of life, and in regarding him as a "little schoolboy", they feel that he will soon be leaving them, and they start to think about separation. Depressive elements emerge, as shown by the sad remark made by one nurse when she introduced me to the new student nurse: "She is clever; she already has her favourite patients, amongst whom is Giacomo; but his mother will be here when he comes out of his cot, we will not be able to hold him in our arms . . . or perhaps just during the night."

The process of separation, during the final part of the child's stay in hospital, often results in the enactment of defence mechanisms by the nurses. The most common one consists in presenting the preterm child with its boyfriend or girlfriend: the nurse carries a baby of the opposite sex in her arms from the lower-dependency room and introduces it to the child as its "boyfriend" or "girlfriend". This grown-up preterm baby's "boyfriend" or "girlfriend" becomes for the nurses the

department's representative in keeping the child whose departure is imminent close to themselves. Engagement is the rite
that precedes marriage, a bond that is expected to last all life
long.

In the case of Giacomo, this "engagement" was mentioned
by his mother during the last observation session before his
discharge (Box 17). In the session that takes place when
Giacomo is 32 weeks and 4 days old, the nurses start saying
good-bye to him. Owing to the maturation of his central nervous system, his sleep is different in quality. He relates to the
incubator in a different way. When he makes a series of movements with his body and limbs, they no longer resemble sharp
jerks; he is no longer passive. He looks more integrated. As
the nurse had said, extubation is synonymous with life for the
child, giving him the opportunity to have relations with
the outside world. Although he has certainly been supported
and helped by his mother at this stage, he himself is the active
protagonist of this separation process ("he knew how to take off
the tubes"). This is experienced by him as a new separation
from the umbilical cord, a new birth. It is interesting to note
another part of this session, when a nurse who was herself a
preterm infant revisits her problems of that time, while also
communicating to me how the emotive experience of caring for
the newborn comes to an end too precociously, and how difficult it is to tolerate the succession of separation experiences.

The child's first organizational patterns:
32–34 weeks

At 34 weeks and 4 days, Giacomo weighs 1.590 kg. I find
him still asleep, his face down and turned a little to the
right side, quiet. He holds his hand in front of his mouth;
he still wears gloves, because "yesterday, again, he pulled
the feeding tube away and his mother found him with his
face flooded with milk. He is a terrible baby", a nurse
reports: "He grimaces, then becomes quiet again. He
always wants a support: he touches the wall with his foot,

BOX 17
Giacomo's girlfriends

As already mentioned, during the child's recovery phase, once it has passed the 32nd week and finds itself in a good state—not only in terms of survival—the nurses introduce the little patient to its "girlfriend" or "boyfriend", as a sort of defence against the depressive pain of separation. It is an attempt to forge an everlasting link between the child and the department. During this phase, the parents may accept and encourage this phantasy; engagement marks something vital and creative in life, so the phantasy can be taken as a sign of confidence in their child's future.

Giacomo's mother seemed to accept this idea, although—as can be seen from the last observation before discharge—she then reported that Giacomo had had "too many girlfriends". In this way she expressed her pain and anxiety about the length of Giacomo's stay in hospital, which seemed to be measured by his requiring so "many girlfriends": unlike Giacomo, all these girlfriends had only minor problems, so they went home before him after short admission periods.

Sometimes the nurses' proposal stirs up a feeling of rivalry between them and the mothers, which manifests itself clearly and intensely. This was the case, for example, with Marco, a child born at 25 weeks and 4 days. When the nurses introduced Marco's girlfriend, his mother stated that no engagement was to be envisaged for Marco, because when he was grown-up he would become either a priest or a monk. This showed her clear desire to appropriate her child entirely to herself: during the period of hospitalization she has not yet had the chance to take full possession of her child, so she totally excludes from her relationship the maternal function of the "department", which has of necessity taken care of her little boy so far.

goes into the corners, then he enjoys being caressed and bathed. He is good, alert, has two enormous eyes", she adds.

Now Giacomo is motionless, quiet, his little arms and legs bent. His right hand is leaning against his face. "He is terrible!" the nurse carries on. Giacomo rapidly moves his limbs. He stretches his shoulders and legs, crouches by lifting his bottom, makes some grimaces and breathes regularly. He seems to smile (reflex smile) in his sleep, moving the toes of his right foot, then finally becomes quiet again. He moves his feet alternately; he crouches by lifting his bottom and sliding to right or left, planting his legs down on the cot. He stretches his arm and then becomes motionless.

On the basis of the data in the observation, to be confirmed by echographic investigations made during his intrauterine life, one wonders whether already (at 32 weeks, certainly by the end of the 34th week) some of the child's organization patterns can be outlined. In Giacomo's case, one of his fundamental organization patterns can be seen in the state of well-being described by the nurse: "He is good, alert, he has two enormous eyes." As previously mentioned, the beginning of wakefulness and the following stabilization of sleep–waking states are very important for the child's mental and physical health (see Boxes 14 and 16). "He is a terrible boy" is a comment on the child's curiosity and vitality, which can also lead him to do dangerous things, such as pulling out the feeding tube and flooding his face with milk.

A second organization pattern can be seen in the child's motility characteristics, which, together with the intense role played by the child's eyes, seem to allow him to experience early introjection and projection processes. The search for contact by means of his little foot, his experimenting with different positions and finding an ideal one (lying across the incubator, with his head against the wall), his tendency to slide around, showing his wish to explore the different corners of the incubator, all indicate his ability and his special way of exploring internal space. These characteristic movements feature his own specific pattern of relating to the inside of the object.

Thought formation:
the integration of sensori-motor experiences and emotional experiences deriving from the object relation

In mummy's arms:
the actual birth;
the establishment of rhythms and mental functioning

The child can usually be taken out of the incubator and carried in its parents' arms from 35 weeks, if its clinical condition is satisfactory. The mother, in particular, can finally fulfil her strong desire to hold her child in her arms, which has been increasing as time goes on. With the nurses' help, she can finally take full care of the child. Now the infant observations take place with the baby in its mother's arms and can provide more meaningful data about the establishment of rhythms and mental mechanisms. It is now possible to observe definitely the formation of mental processes such as introjection, projection, projective identification, and splitting.

Giacomo came out of the incubator at 35 weeks and 3 days. During the session on that day, we see him in his mother's arms ready to be fed. He is looking up towards his mother, but he looks tired . . . the mother is talking to him. It is a particularly intense session, when his mother manages to talk to him about life in a very touching way, showing a high appreciation of beauty and of their relationship: "Today is spring, life is so beautiful . . . but you do not seem to be interested, not even in milk. . . . You know what I'll do, I'll let you have a taste, so you can see whether you'll feel like it afterwards. . . ." She squeezes a few drops of milk from the nipple in his mouth. The child seems particularly lively. His eyes are open, and he is taking notice of what is happening; now he abruptly turns towards the breast and stops there, without sucking.

It looks as though he is listening to what his mother is saying. Then the child grasps her finger, stretches himself out, and then curls up against the breast; then he turns away, holding his hand spread out on the breast. His

BOX 18

Feeding the child:
the tube; taste stimulation;
non-nutritional sucking; the milk feed

The feeding of the preterm newborn is a very important aspect, not only of its physical but also of its psychological care. The naso-gastric tube was reintroduced in our department three and a half years ago, since it can be held in position for up to a month. It has replaced the naso-jejeunal tube, which had been used by us since 1981. The naso-jejeunal tube was chosen then because it could remain in position for up to five days, whereas the naso-gastric tube available at that time had to be removed and re-applied up to ten times a day, giving rise to several problems for the baby, such as vomiting. The new naso-gastric tube, which can stay in place for a whole month, avoids the risk of necrotizing enterocolitis (NEC) incurred by naso-jejeunal feeding.

From the beginning of hospitalization, the baby is offered taste stimulation to try to start it sucking. In our department, we start even before the 28th week (as indicated by Bu'Lock, Woolridge, & Baum) if the baby's condition allows. The nurses place a piece of gauze soaked in sweetened water in the child's mouth and observe it. Usually he appreciates this stimulation very much, and in the words of some nurses is "enraptured", moving his mouth and showing his pleasure. When this happens, the nurses continue with the practice, and eventually offer their little finger or a tiny dummy to the infant. Again the child's response is observed, and if he seems to like it and does not get tired, and the parameters indicating his state of health are favourable (heart-beat, breathing, PO2, PCO2), they persevere with the dummy (Field et al., 1982; Bernbaum, Pereira, Watkins, & Peckham, 1983).

mother explains to me that she does not want to force him; she wants him to enjoy being fed; she does not want him to associate the breast with something that is too tiring or stressful (Box 18). He is now holding the nipple in his mouth.

If the child looks tired, the practice is stopped for the time being. It is the child himself who communicates when it is ready to be fed orally. This is not strictly connected with its gestational age, as every child has its own way of behaving: some become restless, cry, or put their finger in their mouth, indicating a need to be orally fed; others are more weak and listless and need more time to become ready.

A satisfactory and effective milk feed requires the co-ordination of the child's respiratory, sucking, and swallowing abilities (Miller, 1982; Johnson & Salisbury, 1975). This entails the functional interaction of lips, mandibles, maxilla, tongue, pharynx, larynx, and oesophagus. Meier and Anderson (1987) believe that during the earliest stages of development newborns are more competent at breast-feeding than bottle-feeding. A study carried out by Bu'Lock, Woolridge, and Baum (1990) shows that full co-ordination between sucking, breathing, and swallowing is only achieved in children older than 37 weeks of gestation, even though the ability to suck and to swallow is present at 32 weeks. This is not surprising if one remembers that these functions have been gradually developing in the foetus for a long time—starting at the 11th week (Miller, 1982) or even earlier, at 9 weeks (according to Tajani & Ianniruberto, 1990).

For all the above reasons, milk sucking is much more tiring and complicated for the premature child than for the child born at term. We often see the preterm newborn's "failure" in this, and his efforts to implement complex actions aimed at protecting the respiratory tract. Thus, after a few vigorous suckings, the preterm newborn has more prolonged apnoeas than does the baby born on time. The apnoea is then followed by "bursts of breathing", during which the baby prevents the milk from flowing down into his mouth—also using his tongue to block the nipple.

The way his mother describes the child is very poetic, and she gives the impression that this is the way it has to be: suggesting that her way of offering herself to him represents everything that is necessary for him, without tiring him too much. If one examines the sequence more carefully, further details emerge. It can be seen that the mother seems able to perceive through the child's slightest and most subtle movements some sort of message to her, which she shows she understands and respects. So we can see at this level of development what we call "projections" and what Melanie Klein (1946) has defined as "projective identification". The mother is able to understand Giacomo's communications, so she teaches us to grasp this mental capability in the baby.

Giacomo's clinging to his mother's hand here seems to be a fully enjoyable act, different from his grabbing at the sheet of the cot when he was in the incubator. When he stretches himself and curls up against the breast, one has the impression that he is looking for something he likes, rather than doing this because he is afraid. The mother seems to be aware that he is tired and finds it difficult to adjust to life; so, while talking to him, she allows the baby to take all the time he needs in exploring the breast.

> The child makes full use of it: he puts his tongue out and calmly explores his mother's breast, interspersed with long pauses. Then he starts wiggling, and his mother interprets his fidgetiness as hunger. To me, as an observer, it does not seem so. But the intense way Giacomo starts sucking at the nipple shows how through his wiggling the mother somehow understood his needs.

This sequence again demonstrates the mother's great ability to adjust to Giacomo's rhythms, giving him space for pauses in which he nods his little head and says "Eh!", then sucking with rhythmical force (Viola, 1991). We can see how the experience of being understood allows this child to experience a good introjection through sucking rhythmically and nodding. (These features—sucking and nodding—have already been noted by Fornari, 1966, in the context of the introjection of a good object by the baby.)

When the mother takes the nipple out of Giacomo's mouth, he remains quiet, with his eyes closed and his arms stretched out. This sense of full abandonment allows him to stay quietly in his mother's arms and to trust her completely. The first evidence of his dependence emerges at this point. The above sequence makes us wonder about the special way in which this child must experience his relation with the breast, not only because it is a new, unknown object, but also because as such a seriously premature baby, he is learning for the first time to swallow and breathe together. The fatigue that comes over a newborn of this gestational age can be fully understood through this observation. It means that things must be approached gradually, to be fully appreciated. Slowness allows him to savour the new experience of drops of milk dripping down his mouth, his oesophagus, and then his stomach: no longer coming up, but giving him a sensation of fullness and exhaustion at the same time. He makes use of "slowness" to give the necessary time and space to these functions, so they can perform in a fully satisfactory way. It is important for the child to experience the act of swallowing and breathing in a way that is not suffocating. It must not be forgotten that he has had respiratory problems since his birth and throughout his stay in the incubator. His mother follows what her child "tells" her; the propositional competence is very clear here, and the child manifests his pleasure in achieving his own equilibrium. Giacomo clearly seems to have achieved that rhythm of safety that has been described by Tustin (Box 19), and at the same time, the resolution of his suffering.

BOX 19

The safety rhythm

In her book on *Autistic Barriers in Neurotic Patients*, Frances Tustin (1986) deals with the importance of a mutual adjustment between mother and child during breast-feeding, so as to establish a "synchronized" rhythm: this is the result of a balanced harmony between the rhythms of child and mother. According to Tustin, people who were fortunate in their early childhood in enjoying and introjecting the emotional experiences deriving from rhythmical adjustment between mouth and breast (as differentiated from each other) will later be more receptive in their own experience of love relationships as well as of religious and aesthetic ones.

BOX 20
Early mother–infant individuation

This observation is confirmed by Stern (1985), who does not recognize a period of physiological symbiosis during the first moments of life. He states that there is a "limited confusion" between the self and the other, even at the very beginning of life. This observation corresponds to what had been assumed initially by Melanie Klein (1952a, 1952b), who does not refer to any such stage or phase in the child's mental development; she never refers to symbiotic or autistic phases but, rather, to "moments".

This session, then, shows the harmony between mother and child. Their relationship is not founded on fusion or symbiosis, but on a healthy separateness: the mother also talks about her detachment—how she is herself, and the child is not the mother (Box 20).

The mother's depression and its mirror-like repercussions on the nursing staff; the emotional experience modulated by the child

The pirate

As other works have already stressed, depressive experiences are a constant element in the parents of seriously premature infants. Giacomo's mother goes through this as well, just when the condition of the baby is improving. During this period, the child seems to be very lively and peremptorily displays the intensity of his appetite for milk and for the relationship with his mother.

Today he is 36 weeks and 1 day old, and I am observing him while he is having his evening feed. He seems very

lively; he has big eyes; he is clinging to his mother's nipple
and sucking greedily. His mother tells me that he is
playing the pirate, because he is holding his hand over his
left eye; he looks alternately in front of him and then up
towards his mother's eyes. Now he is still, with his mouth
closed, his eyes looking at his mother . . . then he starts
sucking again with a will. He sucks strongly, staring
straight in front of him. He sucks with energy, while
holding his right hand open beneath the nipple, without
touching it. The last fingers of his left hand touch the
breast. He goes on sucking vigorously, looking straight in
front of him. He sucks greedily, then detaches himself
from the breast, his mouth closed and arms relaxed.

We see here the intensity of the child's relation with
the breast, through the physical contact, but mainly through
the action of incorporation—taking the nipple inside by means
of his mouth, and taking in the mother's look by means of
his eyes, while the mother seems to experience this "taking
in" through strong and lively sucking as aggressive, which
she expresses by saying that today Giacomo is acting the
"pirate".

We can try to understand this experience by focusing on the
image of the child screening himself: the "pirate-like" attitude
of covering his eye with his hand, turning his eyes away from
his mother, and looking straight in front of him, lowering his
eyelids, keeping his mouth closed, detaching himself from the
breast, and staying still. All these gestures appear to be a way
of giving a rhythm to this relationship, which seems to be so
intense for him that he can hardly tolerate it. That is why he
gives the impression of adjusting the flow of his intake through
eyes, mouth, and bodily contact. The strength of the emotional
experience seems to convert itself into a state of physical exhaustion. It seems too much for him to take in the bodily
contact, the breast, and his mother's gaze at the same time;
he almost seems frightened and exhausted by it. But when he
realizes that he can still get in touch with this new and still
unfamiliar experience of vitality and strength, he seems to find
pleasure in it, and intersperses his sucking at the breast with a
series of "Eh . . . eh . . . eh's".

At this point, his mother looks tired instead. In fact, in the midst of this vigorous and lively feed, she averts her gaze from her child and starts talking about how tired the nurses look and how lonely and overburdened with work they seem, as a result of the hospital staff cuts. She then refers to the pain and helplessness she has felt for the mother of Sabrina, the young terminally ill patient mentioned in chapter two, with whom she has talked during the night because they are room neighbours. Thus the mother breaks off her interaction with the child once he has overcome his sucking difficulties and shows himself to be particularly full of energy; his emotional needs seem to be too intense for a mother forced to undergo three and a half months of anxiety with a strong commitment to nurture hope "at any cost", and followed now by great tiredness.

From this we can gauge how much mental suffering is involved in tuning in with the needs of such a tiny child, who cannot be stimulated too much but whose need is so intense that his mother feels powerless, like Sabrina's mother (the terminal patient), whom even the most loving care will fail to keep alive. Even though with Giacomo the worry about death has been completely overcome, the inner intensity of the infant now imposes rhythms of perception and response that are so incredibly full of emotional tension that they can become persecutory for the adult. Through the exhaustion and depression of Giacomo's mother it is possible to quantify the degree of mental commitment made by all the staff in the face of fatigue and other difficulties.

Some signs of depression had already emerged amongst the staff in the work group based on the session when Giacomo was 33 weeks and 2 days old and was already showing his vitality and sense of well-being. When the nurses started seeing him as a "grown-up" baby (a "schoolboy"), paying attention to the outside world, they showed they were starting to think about separation. One of them, who had herself been born prematurely, was reconsidering her own situation through the observation of Giacomo: she suggested the emotional involvement with the child comes to an end too suddenly, and it is very difficult to bear the succession of separation experiences. The adults involved in the care of these children feel a continuous urge to enter and re-emerge from identifications (Klein, 1955) with the child and its parents.

The staff need to equip themselves with a complex mental functioning in order to cope with the emotional intensity that these identifications entail. While the child feels the need to screen itself from a flow of emotional sensations so intense they cannot be integrated, the mother and the staff need to oppose a depressive reaction, which could become a defence from such an intense emotional need. It is interesting to note that the mother is affected by depression in the same way as the nurses: that is, she can control it as long as her child is in danger; yet once it is certain that the child is out of danger, this depressive state emerges.

Splitting: the toilet breast; the experience of trusting, of being contained

The last observation of Giacomo at the hospital took place when he was 37 weeks and 4 days old, and about to be discharged. This session is only three days after the previous one, and his mother has already rediscovered the vitality and richness of her emotional resources.

Giacomo is in his mother's arms, ready for his evening feed. He has beautiful big blue eyes; he seems to be smiling; he is looking at his mother, complaining slightly, while turning his head. His mother invites him to have his feed, then she remarks: "He is growing . . . now he doesn't only want to eat." Giacomo is still; he is actually looking at his mother, holding his mouth half-open on the nipple; then, all of a sudden, he turns his mouth and grabs the nipple, sucking voraciously, still holding his left hand in the strange position described before—covering his left eye. His mother talks to him and tells me about the fact that her husband has unfortunately had to go away on business.

In the meantime a nurse arrives, holding a small baby girl. The mother tells me it is Giuliana, Giacomo's "girlfriend", from the cot next to his: "She was so graceful in the incubator, lying on her side . . . Giacomo has had so many girlfriends since he's been here, they have all gone home before him" (see Box 17). Now he is only sucking from time to time, resting for long moments, as though half asleep at the breast. The telephone rings, and the mother wonders whether it is her husband calling to say he has arrived in the place where he will be staying for a week. And, indeed, it is he. The mother goes to the phone with Giacomo in her arms.

During this first part of the session, one is struck by the degree to which Giacomo's mother seems at home in the hospital. She seems so at ease that it is as though she were walking about the rooms of her own house, holding the baby in her arms.

Once she has spoken with her husband on the phone, she comes back into the room. The baby is sleeping at her breast, his head close to the nipple. She sits down, while the child goes on sleeping. He moves his lips from time to time. He is motionless. His mother says to him: "Giacomo, have you finished feeding now?" She lifts him closer to her breast, and he complains. He stays still, with his right cheek on his mother's breast. Then he moves and leans on his left cheek, makes a grimace, moves his head backward, still holding his mouth in front of the nipple, and grumbles. "He's sleepy. . . . I think he has had enough", says his mother, a little worriedly; "however, he's strong, and one side only should be alright for him". After a moment, she says she wants to check whether he is doing this because he is dirty; she stands up, and I assume she is going to change him, so I follow her. Instead, she goes to weigh him and says, "he has had 60 grams". She is out of sight for a while, then I see she is washing the baby, who had indeed dirtied himself, and she comments: "It bothered him." While lying on the changing table, Giacomo has his eyes open and glances at his

mother. She then sits him down to let him burp. He
complains and goes on complaining when lying supine in
her lap, with his arms stretched out and his hands open;
he stays in this position, looking at his mother with his
eyelids half-open, while she is talking to him.

We see that the bodily experience of defecating is experienced in a slightly different way from when he was in the
incubator—when he arched his little bottom because he felt
dirty. Here the gestures of turning his head backward and still
holding his mouth in front of the nipple suggest that he is
associating the bothering dirty feeling with the breast, and we
can see some possible confusion between the dirty nappy and
the breast, as though the fact of being bothered by his dirty
bottom is caused by the breast, which is disturbing him,
becoming the "toilet breast". His mother understands his message and cleans his bottom.

It is very interesting to note how the baby glances at his
mother after this. Here it is possible to perceive the splitting by
the child between the toilet breast and the feeding breast: even
after being cleaned, he still seems unsure and confused and
carries on complaining a little bit; then he becomes willing to
look at his mother again and listen to her, with his arms open
and hands outstretched, in such an attitude of abandonment
that it makes his mother slightly anxious. Giacomo's capacity
for abandonment, which has been observed on various
occasions, testifies to the child's trustful experience of being
contained.

Conclusions

The regular observation of a seriously preterm newborn, as
exemplified by the case of Giacomo, was found to be extremely
valuable. As I had hoped, it allowed us to follow the development of the child's mental dynamics at embryonic level,
becoming ever more complex as time progressed. These were:
early object differentiation; introjective processes; projective
identification; splitting and dependence. The observation experience not only traced these phenomena but also pointed out

the great difficulty of the mental work undertaken by the medical and non-medical staff when caring for these children. Initially there is the confrontation with death, and then the non-linear evolution of the relationship with life—a highly complex operation analogous to the newborn's own non-linear development—which may become blocked at any time.

Owing to the observation work, we learned to become aware of our own defence mechanisms, which emerge whenever we are faced with delicate and complex situations for which we are not automatically adequately equipped. Sometimes we are powerless to deal with the extremity of need that confronts us, as in the case of Sabrina, the little terminal patient, and her mother.

Through the discussion on the observation material in the work group it became clear that the first difficulty in observation consists in being swamped by overwhelming anxiety. The second difficulty is the need to continuously enter into and then emerge from the identification with "the other" (parents or child), and then both when the child starts to improve and it is ready for discharge and when the child unfortunately does not survive the necessary premature interruption of the emotional experience of caring and the preparation for separation need. With reference to mental processes, these difficulties have been identified by underlining the different characteristics in thought of the people surrounding the child. In the discussions of the observation material within the work group, the different ways of considering the problem and dealing with the child during its life in hospital came out.

What, then, is the function of the observation? Firstly, it is essential for the observer to experience personally how difficult it is to think about the child under certain conditions. He comes across paralysing experiences. The identification with the newborn points out the lack of mental competence in the adult and calls for a step forward to meet these new demands. It is important to examine and discuss this in the work group, for the observer's function is to make people think about the problem and become aware of its complexity. This has led to changes in the nurses' way of thinking (Box 21), in the setting of the observation, in my neuropsychological evaluation of the child, and in the interview procedures with parents.

BOX 21

The change in the nurses

As already stated in the text, the observation work has resulted in a change in the nurses' way of thinking.

What does this change actually consist of? According to them, it is something different from what usually occurs after reading a text or attending a conference. It is due not only to material in the observations verifying how the child has responded to their actions, but derives also from the fact of "being fully involved in everything concerning the baby". The head-nurse says:

"It is one thing to listen to psychologists—you can either believe them or not; if, for example, they explain the importance of caressing the child before the bronchial suctioning, you may follow their advice, but it is another matter to observe the baby yourself and try to understand what, in your opinion, is the best posture for it to be in when this is done. But that is not all. At that moment, you also understand what the manipulation means, both for the one who makes it and for the baby who receives it [Long, Philip, & Lucey, 1980]. You understand the kind of relationship that is established between you and the baby at that moment, and you can observe what its response is. Then what has happened between yourself and the child can be understood even more deeply if it is examined with other colleagues in the work group during the weekly discussions."

The nurse, through her example, wants to express that the change in the group is really a result of the nurses' different attitude: of their greater open-mindedness in perceiving the emotional experience surrounding the baby. They are more receptive but also more aware of the emotions, without being overwhelmed by them. This implies the ability to enter in and come out from different identifications with parents and child. The head nurse lets us understand that the change in the group is essentially a new way of learning—what Bion (1962) has defined as "learning from the emotional experience".

During Giacomo's first observation sessions, the child was often sleeping. After a while I would find one or both parents near the incubator and then one of the nurses present in the department would come close to it. Sessions of very special interest took place in which I was present as silent observer, while both parents or just the mother talked with the nurse about the child. This experience of observation, characterized by the nurses' lively comments, made me think how useful it would be to offer the group the opportunity to observe the personality development of each newborn present in the department more often and systematically. This was how we decided to hold a weekly meeting with the nurses in the room where the most seriously preterm or most at risk newborn's incubator was located. The group would sit around the newborn in the incubator, in an "open-door" situation (for more detail, see chapter two). I played the role of leader and, using my particular experience in observation, guided the group members to focus their attention on observing the child. If someone uses language indiscriminately, it is up to the leader to act cautiously as a mediator.

It was possible to see that in this situation nurses, without their nursing duties being distracted in any way, could anticipate the emergence of vital features in even the most seriously premature newborn, even from the first moments of its admission (Box 22). Their way of thinking about the child was changed remarkably: before this, the group had always maintained clear-cut distinctions between the existential condition of the preterm and the full-term child. The possibility of the preterm newborn feeling pain was not recognized: thus their shivering was not seen as a manifestation of pain but as a characteristic of their gestational age. Likewise, a clear-cut distinction was made between the suffering for the death of a full-term infant and that of a preterm newborn, the latter usually being denied. Through the "open-door" observation of the newborn in the incubator, the staff learned to attach more importance to their own observations about the infant. They became more aware of the significance of their own actions, which were no longer seen as merely an accessory to the mechanical equipment or to the drug treatment prescribed by the medical staff, but as complementary to these and equally

BOX 22

The first "open-door" observation

The first "open-door" observation of Marta is given below, as an example:

The group sits around the baby girl, who was born before the 25th week, weighing 820 g; together with me, they make the first direct observation of the baby girl. She was admitted to our department two days earlier. Only her face can be seen, since owing to thermoregulation problems, she is lying on the lamb's fleece and is protected by a plastic cover.

She is motionless. I comment on her fine, delicate features, but also on the jelly-like transparency of her face, which reminds us of the pictures in embryology texts.

The present neonatologist is pessimistic about her chances of survival, owing to her gestational age and to the transportation conditions when she was transferred from the hospital where she was born to our department.

The nurses present, however, do not agree with him: "We believe she will make it, because when she arrived here she was nice-looking, rosy, very lively, despite being transferred without the respirator. She was active, shrieking, rejected the respirator, then she needed to be soothed."

This session was completely different from what had happened during the discussion of the first observation of Giacomo. That occasion had resulted in silence from the group. Then my attempts to evoke interest received responses such as: "Well, what do you expect, at levels like these we cannot see the child . . . we're just interested in the proper functioning of the respirator, the right heart-beat", and so on.

necessary for the child's well-being and growth—in particular, its emotional development. This new awareness meant that more appropriate actions could be made on the child's behalf, defined as "preventive environmental actions". However tiny, immobile, and unresponsive the newborn may be, it is fulfilling to try to understand and meet its needs. It is then satisfying to see these efforts rewarded in the infant's growth and well-being. Recognizing that the infant has a mental life serves as a further stimulus towards greater attention and interest in the child, thus leading to an improvement in its care.

The observation experience also affected the development of my neuropsychological evaluation of the young patient and my meetings with the parents. Originally my evaluation of the child was made only just before its discharge, in its parents' presence. Interviews were held with them during its hospitalization, but separately from their child. My experience with Giacomo's parents near the incubator, from the first moments of his life, showed me how meaningful it was for the parents to make contact and to be informed about the child's neurological development even from the early stages, when their anxiety may interpret the peculiar reactions of the child as a sign of suffering even when it is a normal characteristic of that gestational age (Box 23).

This was why I decided to carry out the child's neuropsychological development evaluations from the beginning of hospitalization during two or three weekly meetings with the parents near the child's incubator. I listened to their comments, answered them, then described and remarked on what the child was doing at that moment, emphasizing the aspects that were most significant in terms of the child's recovery. I also explained the nature of some of the critical moments that might occur during its hospitalization, to help them to understand these better and tolerate them without undue anxiety.

The data that emerged from the infant observations made together with the parents and from the "open-door" observation carried out with the nurses' group allowed me to make up a picture outlining the child's specific "propositional and interactive competence". My thinking about this, which was communicated to the parents as well as to the nurses, had a stimulating effect; in consequence, their own observation skills improved, and they discovered new elements and details which contributed to a much richer and more complete picture of the child's emerging physiognomy and identity. (Chapter one deals more specifically with the meaning that this new intervention has for the parents. It does not replace but integrates previous

---

BOX 23

The child's abrupt starting; active sleep

From the 29th to the 32nd weeks, the child spends most of its time in an "active" sleep, characterized by sudden, rough motor movements, followed by grimaces, eyelid contractions, etc. The parents are often worried by the child's behaviour and interpret it as an expression of serious malaise.

---

arrangements—the interviews with parents and the child's neuropsychological evaluation before discharge from hospital.)

The changes in the group's way of thinking and in the methodology of the therapeutic actions are a direct consequence of the observation work. The fact of a doctor simply standing near the incubator, looking at the tiny child inside it but refraining from stating or planning anything, indicates that here is a phenomenon that is still to be fully explored and understood, because so far very little is known about it. In this way the observer conveys to the group a pre-verbal message of astonishment and of admiration for this phenomenon. And the preterm newborn within the neonatal intensive care unit comes to be regarded with the hope and respect of an event whose features are waiting to be fully revealed.

CHAPTER FOUR

The neuropsychological
screening of the infant
before its discharge from hospital

The neuropsychological screening of the infant, in addition to a neurological examination, is carried out only when the infant is in the lower-dependency room, or when it has reached term and its discharge is imminent. During the earlier phases of hospitalization (for reasons explained in chapter three, and in particular in Box 5), the assessment of neurological maturation and of possible nervous system distress is performed through infant observation. The clinical examination is compared with the functional activities of the nervous system and morphological elements resulting from examinations such as the EEG and ultrasound, performed on the newborn in the standard manner (Couchard, De Bethmann, & Sciot, 1982).

The neuropsychological screening of the preterm newborn—and of newborn infants generally, especially during the first stage—is based on observation, as outlined and illustrated in this chapter. This approach is in line with indications given at present by the major European and American schools (Cioni & Prechtl, 1988; Korner et al., 1987; Milani Comparetti, 1982b; Prechtl, 1984; Touwen, 1990). The above-mentioned researchers attach great importance to the newborn's variability of movement and its spontaneous motility (on which depends its "propositional competence"). Echographic (ultrasound) studies of foetal motility have influenced researchers considerably, especially those with a neurological background (Cioni & Prechtl, 1988; Cioni et al., 1988; Milani Comparetti, 1982a; Prechtl, 1984; Touwen, 1990), by attaching greater importance to observation in studies of the newborn. Findings based on echographic observations have notably reduced the significance given to the role of the archaic reflexology, which used to predominate in infant screening before echography was discovered (Peiper, 1961; Saint-Anne Dargassies, 1974; Thomas & Autgaerden, 1966; Vojta, 1974).

The neuropsychological screening of the infant before its discharge is carried out in the presence of its parents and of the nurses who have taken care of it in hospital. In my view it is a very meaningful event. It serves as a catalyst for all the previous preventative activities described in this study. I also attach a therapeutic significance to this screening, calling the parents' attention to the child's most vital aspects and positive features in terms of a culmination of our collective knowledge so far (nurses, parents, and myself), when we were observing the infant's behaviour in the incubator.

I stress the importance of holding the child, of making eye-contact, of talking. This helps to identify the anxieties derived from the suffering the baby has experienced, in particular because of illness, loneliness, and traumatic medical procedures.

At this point, I explain the reasons for the possible fear the child may have later when getting undressed or when touched on its feet or head—the so-called "little-hat phobia". During the examination, I explain to parents the meaning of possible shivering, psychogenic hypertonia, or states of irritability. I also explain the point of the follow-up meetings after discharge from hospital. In cases of serious neurological impairment, requiring the immediate start of a rehabilitation programme (see chapter eight), the physiotherapist who will be responsible for following the child will be introduced to the parents in the ward, before discharge.

Infant examination

In my neurological evaluation I attach great importance to the state of consciousness of the infant (in line with Brazelton, 1973, 1984, Korner et al., 1988, Tronick et al., 1990, etc.), as already mentioned in chapter three (Box 16). The meaning of its responses to stimuli strongly depends on its state of consciousness, and this must be taken into account when interpreting them. The degree of deliberation in its reactions to internal and external stimuli is an important factor in gauging its potential ability for self-control (Brazelton, 1973). During the neurological screening, it is important to consider the state change model and the direction and stability of response to internal and external stimuli. The criteria defining the state of consciousness are based on the studies by Prechtl and Beintema (1964), Wolff (1966), Brazelton (1973, 1984), and Korner et al. (1988).

In my own neurological screening of the infant, I have taken into account the works of major authors such as Amiel-Tison and Grenier (1980), Thomas and Autgaerden (1966), Benedetti, Ottaviano, Galletti, and Gagliasso (1982), Bollea, (1964), Brazelton (1973, 1984), Grisoni Colli (1968), Lilli and Victor Dubowitz (1981), Egan, Illingworth, and MacKeith (1969), Illingworth (1966), Korner et al. (1987), Le Métayer (1989), Milani Comparetti and Gidoni (1976), Paine (1960), Paine et al. (1964), Peiper (1961), Prechtl and Beintema (1964), Saint-Anne Dargassies (1972, 1974), Sheridan (1977), Vojta (1974), and Volpe (1987). Knowledge of the work of the above authors is, in my opinion, of fundamental importance in identifying the infant's potential for neurological evolution, and in recognizing deviations in time. This is the context in which, together with my own clinical experience, I have devised the programme of infant screening that I use.

As already mentioned, it is important to examine the infant's state of consciousness, and to do this in the quietest possible conditions. It is recommended that an infant born at term should be examined three days after birth, in a quiet room, sufficiently warm, between feeding times, etc. The child should be handled very carefully to achieve its best performance. It is necessary to be as cautious and delicate as possible

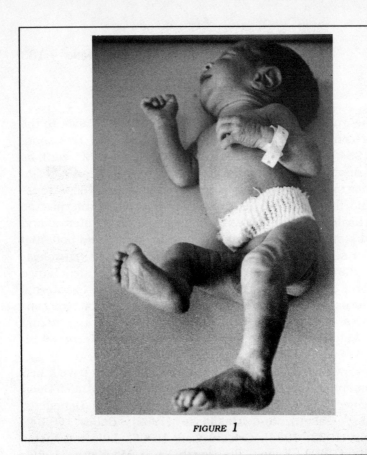

FIGURE 1

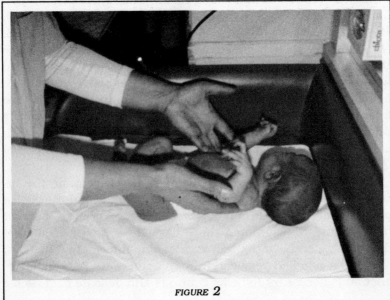

FIGURE 2

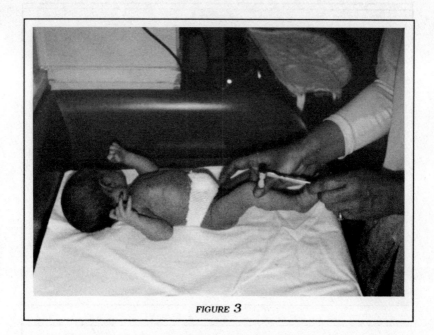

FIGURE *3*

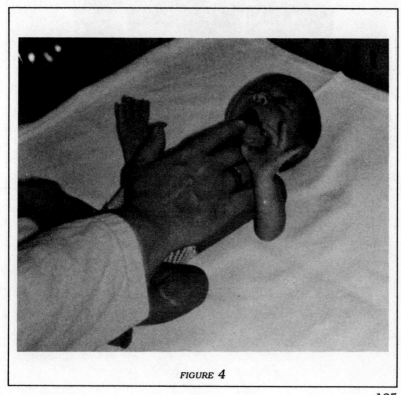

FIGURE *4*

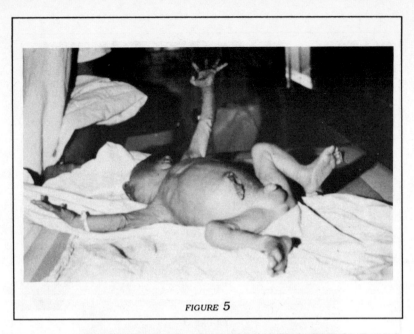

FIGURE 5

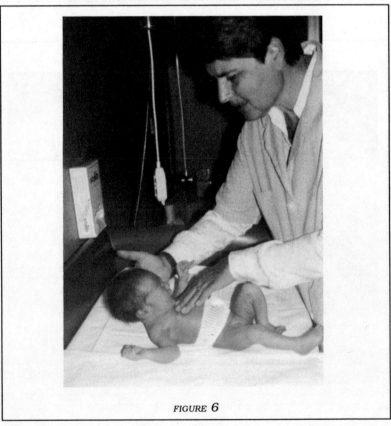

FIGURE 6

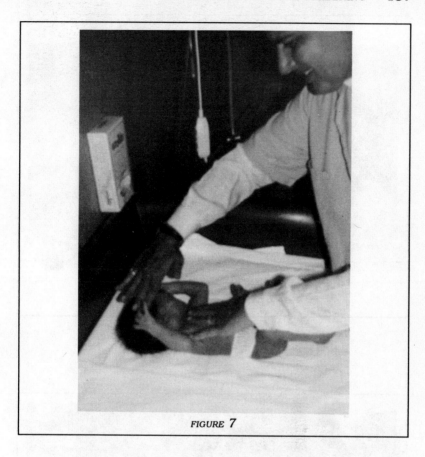

FIGURE 7

and to examine the child when it is awake, attentive, and not crying. Minimal interference when handling the child will allow for a better evaluation of the child's tone and spontaneous activity.

At first, the clothed child is observed supine on the visiting table. Its positions and attitudes as well as its responses to visual and auditory stimuli are observed. Then it is undressed and its reaction to this procedure is observed (Figure 1). Its tone (Figure 2), osteotendinous reflex responses (Figure 3), and the following archaic reflexes are evaluated: rooting response (Figure 4), Moro reflex (Figure 5), symmetric (Figure 6) and asymmetric tonic reflex (Figure 7), and the foot (Figure 8) and hand grasp (Figure 9).

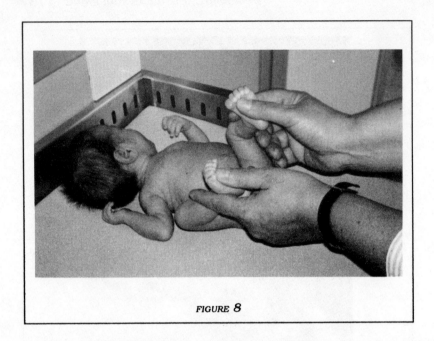

FIGURE 8

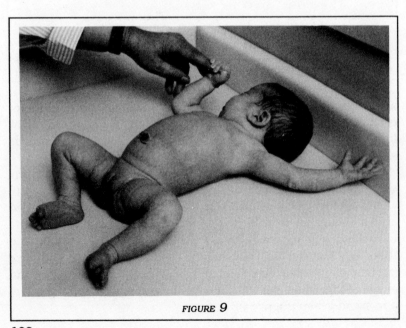

FIGURE 9

138

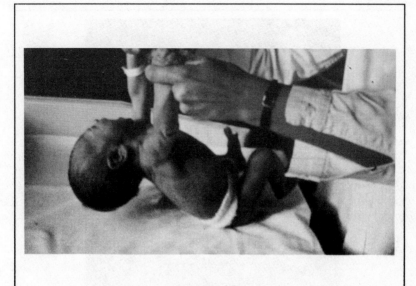

FIGURE *10*

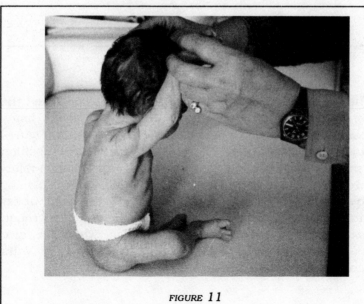

FIGURE *11*

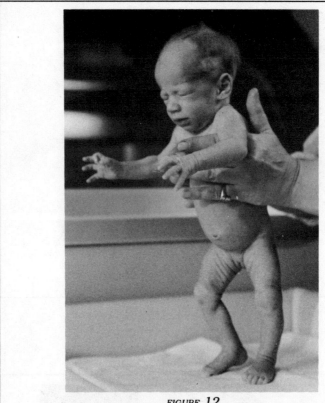

FIGURE 12

Then the child is pulled up into a sitting position, and the responses of its head, trunk, and upper and lower limbs are carefully examined to assess the state of tension (Figures 10 and 11). I then place the child in an upright position and examine the standing (Thomas static straightening) reflex (Figure 12), the automatic walking (Figure 13), and the placing reaction (Figure 14). I delicately lift the infant, holding it under the armpits (Figure 15), and examine the trunk tone through suspension in left and right lateral position, which has also been adopted by Vojta (1974) and defined by him as the "Vojta position reflex" (Figure 16).

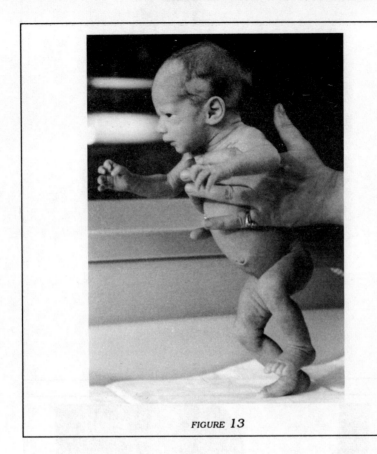

FIGURE 13

Finally, I place the infant in a prone position and examine its postural responses to this (Figure 17). The assessment implemented is similar to the one adopted by the French school (Saint-Anne Dargassies, 1972, 1974; Thomas & Autgaerden, 1966) and to that followed by the Bobaths (1979, pp. 75–107) in their infant assessment.

Normally I would carry out no other examinations, unless some neurological risks emerged from the screening. In that case, according to the findings, I would carry out the specific manoeuvres indicated by the Bobaths (B. Bobath, 1971a, 1971b; K. Bobath, 1980) and by Vojta (1974) in their assess-

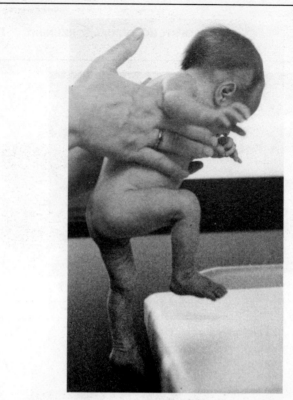

FIGURE 14

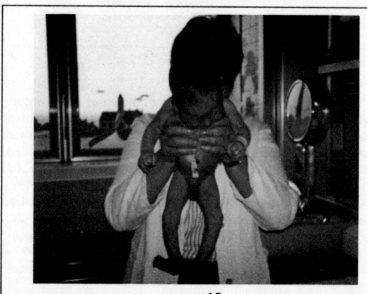

FIGURE 15

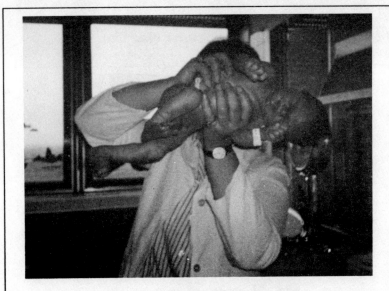

FIGURE 16

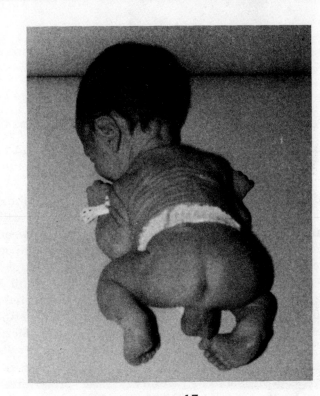

FIGURE 17

143

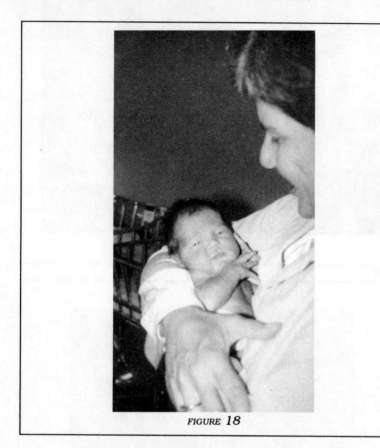

FIGURE 18

ment of the brain-damaged child. As already stated, the child must be handled carefully, in order not to interfere with its spontaneous motility and tone; so I put my finger between the child and the little hammer (as shown in the picture) to obtain the osteotendinous reflex responses (see Figure 3).

I do not intentionally produce any nociceptive stimuli, but I assess the child's ability to soothe itself and to be quieted after being undressed, back in the supine position, after disturbing stimulations have been carried out such as the "Moro response" and the symmetric and asymmetric tonic reflex. I observe the child's ability to console itself, but if it does not, I intervene with soothing actions. (These procedures are described by Brazelton, 1973, 1984, in discussions on infant

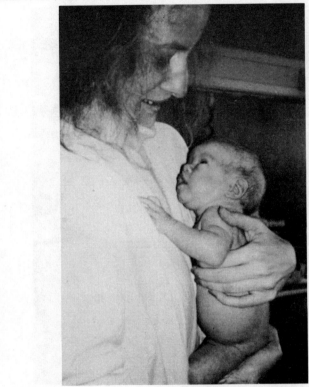

FIGURE 19

consolability in his books. He suggests that the assessment be carried out through increasingly more complex stages: At first, the examiner should confine himself to talking to the child; then he should place a hand on its tummy; then arrange its arms along the midline. If this does not calm the baby, the examiner should pick it up and hold it in his arms, rocking it and offering the dummy. This American author awards different scores on the basis of the level of intervention necessary to console the infant. The newborn's performance here is put into relation with relevant pre- and perinatal factors. In my opinion, not enough stress is put on the difference between the term newborn who is hospitalized for some mild problem, and the seriously premature newborn.) I try to establish eye-contact; I

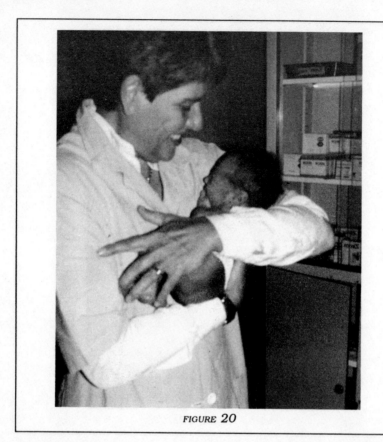

FIGURE 20

talk and touch the baby, and, if this is still not enough, I hold the baby in my arms while whispering into its ears. Sometimes my intervention can bring the child a good degree of consolation (Figure 18), but very often it attains this only if it is held in the arms of its mother (Figure 19). This shows the newborn's very early ability to recognize its mother—a factor mainly linked to the senses of smell and hearing, which have already been in use for several months *in utero*. In my opinion the consolability of the infant, which is also reached through the mother's intervention, has very favourable prognostic implications for its emotional stability in its future life.

Whether the child is soothed with little effort or whether it needs to be held in one's arms, after assessing its

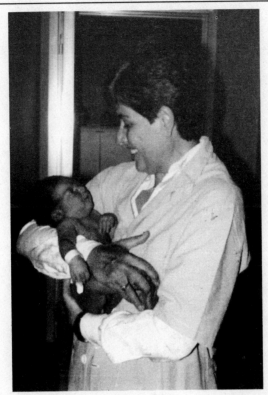

FIGURE 21

"consolability" level I end my neuropsychological screening by
holding the child in my arms. In this way I can assess what
Brazelton (1973, 1984) defines as "cuddliness"—namely, the
newborn's ability to curl up, mould itself, and relax in the
cavity between the examiner's arms, chest, and shoulders (Figure 20). I attach a favourable prognosis to the child's readiness
to accept and enjoy its dependence on the adult. The relationship potential is developed even further if the child tries to
grasp and cling to the examiner, putting its open hand on the
chest and turning its eyes towards the examiner's eyes (Figure
21). This indicates the infant's effort to discover and understand the source of his feeling of contentment.

CHAPTER FIVE

Post-discharge follow-up

The first consultation after the child's discharge from hospital usually takes place at the age of 2 months (actual age) for babies born at term, and at the corrected age of 2 months for babies born prematurely. It is important to leave a certain period after discharge so parents have time to establish an intimate relationship with their child, based on direct mutual knowledge, without the specialist's mediation interfering with it. Sometimes, however, there may be reasons (related to child or parents) for arranging a consultation soon after discharge; likewise parents, if they feel the need, may ask the therapist to bring the consultation forward.

Intervention methodology

Parents are invited to sit in front of the desk where some toys have been laid out, with their child in their arms. I try to make them feel at ease, and I observe the child while the parents talk to me about it (Figure 22).

149

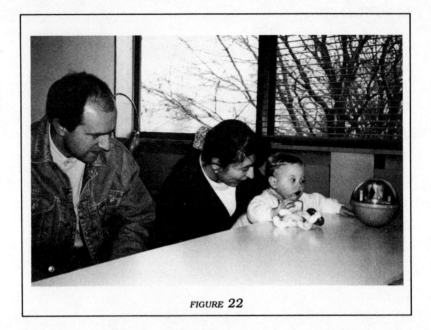

FIGURE 22

It is important to observe how the parent—usually the mother—holds the child, and how the child, while being held, uses its organs of perception and performs movements to relate to the environment (through "free motility" in the phrase of Amiel-Tison and Grenier, 1980). The child is still at an age when its movements show residual philogenetic features. There is a marked latency period in humans between birth and the maturation of the neuronal and functional adjustments appropriate to the extrauterine condition, which only start to operate after the second or third month. During this period the child is in many ways incompetent and responds inadequately even to plain and simple requests from the extrauterine environment. This phenomenon is less marked in other species of primates and seems to stress further the importance of the mother's role in the development of the human infant. It affects the meaning of the sensuous physical contact with the mother through acoustic and visual stimulation, touch, movement, smell (in the animal world, for example, the mother sheep accepts its lamb only after recognizing its smell—see Hafez, 1975). This contact cannot be considered only as the most suitable means of facilitating motor integration and development, but must also be seen as part of a wider function of welcoming and understanding the emotional communications that are the foundation for symbol formation, thinking, and the integration of the self by the child.

After observing the child and exploring its relational attitudes and functions with its parents, I ask the mother to lay the baby down on the neurological examination table and to undress it (Figure 23). I ask parents to do this with children aged no more than 7 or 8 months. This procedure is an important part of the consultation because the mother, left alone with her child, finds a space in which to relate intimately with it. Thus it

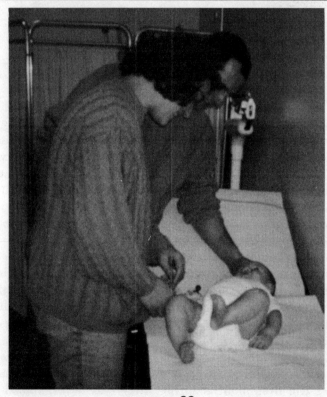

FIGURE 23

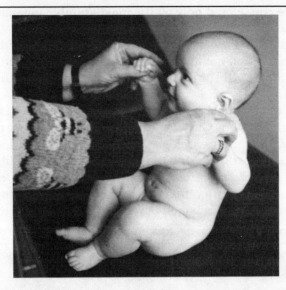

FIGURE 24

is possible for me to observe her manner of handling and talking to it while undressing it—whether she is confident, nervous, intimate, hesitant. At the same time I can observe the child's response. Once the child is undressed, I carry out a neurological examination to assess its development (Figure 24) in the same manner as the pre-discharge assessment: supine, pulled to sitting position, standing, suspended under the arm-pits, Vojta position reflex, prone (see Figures 1 to 17).

For children of 7 or 8 months or more who are able to sit in a stable position, the neurological examination is no longer carried out on the table, as the child might be frightened. I prefer to carry out the evaluation of its spontaneous motility on a mattress on the floor, where a few toys have been placed (Figures 25a and 25b).

The consultations do not follow a set programme. Usually they are more frequent for seriously preterm newborns and during the first months of life; they can be organized on a monthly, fortnightly, or even weekly basis, if risk situations are identified in the child or parents. When the child's development is satisfactory—as in the case of most 8-month-old children—meetings may be held only every three to six months. By this stage the mother may prove to be so confident in her intimate relationship with the child that she facilitates the separation process.

During the follow-up meetings I consider it very useful to explore the way in which parents have worked through and overcome the problem of such a traumatic birth. I give them plenty of space for recalling their feelings about the premature or pathological arrival of their child. I noticed that during the meeting immediately following the birth of the child, the fathers generally preferred to stand back and allow their wife to express her pain and anxiety. Only during the follow-up meetings, when the child's health is satisfactory, does the father fulfil his need to relive his experience of that time. For example, Camilla was a 7-month newborn with a hare-lip, cleft palate, and left lateral cerebral ventricular enlargement, with epileptic seizures. When she was 2 years and 6 months old, her father felt the need to evoke again what he had felt during the period after her birth. Only when the child's development was proving to be satisfactory—despite significant problems—could the father express in abundant detail his experience of parenthood from the moment of his first awareness of the malformations (during the prenatal period), through the birth and the intensely anxious search for a plastic surgeon, to the series of operations and hospital admissions. During this follow-up session he also communicated his desire to write down his experiences, and asked me whether I thought it could be useful for parents with similar problems.

It seems to me that the traumatic experience undergone by these parents can be worked through and overcome if, in response to precise questions asked by me, they say they have not continued to have recurrent distressing dreams in which the child always appears to be in some dangerous situation, and if their child's long period in hospital feels as though it took place a long time ago—a distant memory; also if, as often happens, they tell me they are thinking positively about having another baby.

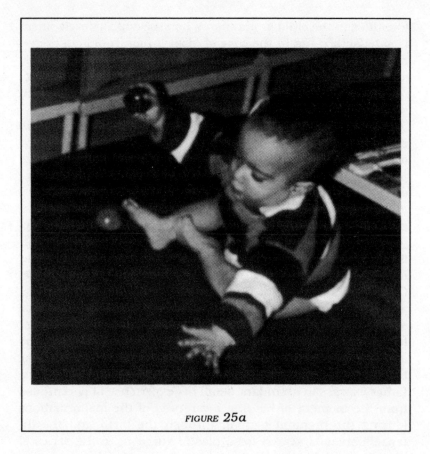

FIGURE 25a

I consider, therefore, that the separation–individuation process is very significant. I evaluate this at the end of the first
year, by observing the way in which the child plays and starts
to walk. I always ask parents whether the child constantly
demands their presence at home, or whether they think it can
stay and play alone for a few minutes while they are in another
room. If the separation experience seems to be satisfactory,
and if no other major problems arise concerning the child or
the parents, I suggest seeing the child once a year up to the end
of the first year of nursery school, and I ask to see all the
drawings the child has made during the year.

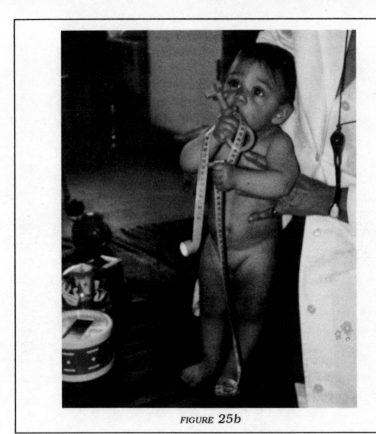

FIGURE 25b

In fact, parents often prefer to have check-ups every six months; in the case of seriously preterm infants, these usually continue until the age of 4 years. I have noticed that with one or two exceptions, the parents become increasingly interested in the way in which the consultations are carried out. The meeting is regarded as an opportunity to take note and discuss various aspects of the child; parents are helped to find the most suitable solutions. The specialist helps them to reflect more thoroughly on the child's problems and qualities, commenting on these features as they emerge during the meeting from the child's play activity.

CHAPTER SIX

Psychopathological conditions

Psychopathological risks

As already stressed in chapter three, the early life of the seriously preterm newborn or of the pathological newborn is characterized, on the one hand, by hyperstimulation and, on the other, by serious sensorial and affective deficiencies. According to Meltzer (1992), this condition can invite the onset of claustrophobic anxieties as well as of major psychopathological states.

Claustrophobic anxieties

Isolation and the absence of contact can correspond for the newborn to the claustrophobic anxiety of being thrown out or thrown away; while the physical hyperstimulation can correspond to the equally painful experience of being closeted in a very narrow environment, from which the newborn derives no comfort and which it does not understand but feels as constraining, crushing, and oppressive. According to Meltzer (1992), the appearance of claustrophobic anxieties—dreadful experiences, which lead to a delusional system—is a risk both for newborns inside the incubator and for adopted children, even if they are just a few weeks old.

After an initial period characterized by isolation, lack of affection, and of the breast relation, the preterm newborn—like the adopted child—finally encounters a woman (the true or new mother) who is eager for a close affectionate bond. The woman can still establish a very close physical relationship with the child, even without the experience of the breast relationship, by encouraging the pauses and spaces necessary for the arrangement of suitable rhythms for the child's development (Tustin, 1986; Viola, 1991). This relationship is "encapsulated" rather than being integrated through breast-feeding.

If one considers how this first life experience of birth (Meltzer & Harris, 1985) becomes an internal model for analogous experiences occurring later in one's life (entry to nursery school, the end of an analysis, etc.), then its vital importance can be understood.

Semiological elements: alarm symptoms

FROM A NEUROLOGICAL INTERPRETATION
OF "SOFT SIGNS"
TO A PSYCHOPATHOLOGICAL INTERPRETATION

In the field of neonatal neurology the importance of the early detection of signs of suffering in the brain has rightly been stressed. Treatment must be as timely as possible because even if it cannot completely repair the damaged nervous system, it can at least reduce the functional damage associated with the injury and guarantee the newborn's development (Bobath, 1967; Negri, 1982, 1983a; Touwen, 1989). For this reason, in infant neurology several semiological elements are taken into consideration during the neonatal period and early infancy, because in some cases they can define true syndromes (see Table 1, page 2, and Table 2, page 5) (see also Touwen, 1989).

Nevertheless, for diagnostic purposes these findings cannot be interpreted strictly neurologically: as Touwen clearly states, in a study of 161 newborns manifesting these signs, only 10% developed cerebral palsy. The author concludes that "not all the early signs eventually turn into a cerebral palsy and that identical signs may show different prognoses; therefore the presence of a syndrome is not necessarily an indication of a neurological disorder."

It is clear that many of the syndromes thus described—the hyperexciteability syndrome, apathetic syndrome, transient dystonic syndrome, irritability, hypo-reactivity, tremor, different types of crying, sleep disorders, etc.—would be left without a proper interpretation if the significance of mental functions were not considered. These operate already in intrauterine life, as evidenced in the fields of psychoanalysis (Bion, 1978; Corominas, 1983a, 1983b; Del Carlo Giannini, 1982; Freud, 1925; Isaacs, 1948; Meltzer, 1986), neurophysiology (Dreyfus-Brisac, 1968; 1970; Jouvet, 1978; Mancia, 1980), and, more recently, in ecographic studies (Ianniruberto & Tajani, 1990; Negri et al., 1990; Prechtl, 1984). The recognition of mental functions is still difficult in the paediatric environment, because at the beginning of life biology does not allow us to differentiate between somatic and psychic functions: "The newborn feels with its body and uses it to express itself" (Negri, 1983b).

The newborn avails itself of all its physical potential and activity to express deep and intense emotions. It is important to recognize the newborn's tendency to experience the emotions of joy or suffering, well-being, discomfort, and uneasiness through bodily sensations. Hence neurologists talk about the extreme variability of muscular tone—which, for the neonate, is then not only a sign of postural attitude. This has been confirmed by the infant observation experience and has led to the recognition of the variability and flexibility of the newborn's posture in response to the behaviour of the mother.

Yet in a newborn at risk of developing cerebral palsy or any other type of psychopathology, postural variability and flexibility are missing, and the child is under the strain of excessive anxiety, which may trigger defence mechanisms. The latter can be manifested as stereotypes and oppose the consensual integration of sense organs.

The child at risk of developing a type of psychopathology is generally one who has spent the first period of its life in an incubator or is constitutionally lacking in a drive for integration. In the child affected by cerebral palsy, the anxiety preceding the appearance of the neurological disorder is due to the disorder itself, which causes suffering in the nervous system (which we can understand by thinking how neurological maturation develops a containing function for primitive anxieties). It is also due to hospitalization in a very traumatizing environment, being isolated in the incubator and still undergoing invasive intervention procedures.

The child at risk can manifest mental operations with pathological features at very early stages of its mental development. I have identified from my experience a whole range of features that may be defined as *alarm symptoms*, since they indicate a psychopathological risk. These "alarm symptoms" are also present in healthy children, yet to a lesser degree; whereas they are widely present in the children at risk. Also, while they appear in a transitional way in healthy children, in children at risk they become predominant and are crystallized parts of the personality, often repeated by the child.

The loss of variability is often the first or one of the first distinctive signs of the disorder: there may be an increase of stereotypy, a reduced adaptability, resulting in a decrease in the ability to interact adequately with the environment, to "cope". The concept of variability, as contrasted with stereotypy, is a very useful instrument for differentiating between normal and deviating functions in the early analysis of the development disorder (Touwen, 1989). It means that here the "alarm symptoms" are so predominant that they oppose the consensual integration of the child's sense organs or sensory capacity. For the sensory components need to integrate: they seek a state of equilibrium, placing themselves in a harmonious relation, which finds its cohesion through the newborn's relation with the mother (who during the early levels of development embodies its satisfied needs).

All these questions about the condition of the child find their expression and answer in the process of infant observation.

During her first session of observation, Francesca, a 10-day-old healthy infant, is happily breast-feeding in her mother's arms. The action is accompanied by the baby's hand opening, closing, and then grasping at the mother's hand, which is supporting and offering the breast. In this satisfactory feeding experience, the oral activity is enriched by another component—the hand grasp, which becomes integrated with the mouth function. In addition, while the mother is feeding the child, she also talks to her. The sucking experience, when it is associated with the mother's voice, is so pleasurable that eventually the little girl turns her eyes up towards the source of her pleasure and stares at her mother while listening and sucking. Thus the function of the sense organs is further enlarged, as they act not separately but in unison—mouth, hand, hearing, sight—to achieve a full integration.

Only when the sense organs remain integrated can pathology be averted. Starting with sense integration at this level of development, the infant passes on to the integrated perception of the other person—usually the mother. We note that at only 10 days old, Francesca pays attention to her mother. According to Meltzer (Meltzer et al., 1975), attention is envisaged "as the strings which hold the senses together in consensuality" (p. 13).

The visual contact with the mother's eyes is a strongly emotional experience for the newborn, in the context of what Meltzer (Meltzer & Harris Williams, 1988) has described as the "aesthetic conflict". This leads the newborn to the perception and introjection of the person as a whole, attracted towards this by a primitive impulsive love, as clearly indicated by the child's smile (Robson, 1967). Sight, therefore, plays a very integrating role in the healthy newborn. Conversely, sight can be used to avert the experience if the child is faced with too painful sensations: it can use its eyes to control or to fix its gaze adhesively to objects. In a situation like this the child is visibly persecuted by catastrophic, paranoid, and confusional anxieties, which may lead to a persistent condition of auto-sensory limitation. The child can be assisted in overcoming these anxieties by a relationship with a person who can help it make differentiations.

In following both healthy infants and those with psychopathological disorders over the past few years, Genevieve Haag (1988) has stressed the importance of contact with the baby's back and nape of the neck, and their connection with introjective organs such as the mouth, the nipple, and above all the eyes, during the newborn's early development. This contact is the first "psychic skin" and is of fundamental importance for the organization of identifications, for the body image, and for the baby's orientation in space. The mother's arms and hands and other support planes sustain the baby's back and neck when it is held and changed. The sensori-motor stimulants felt by the child in these circumstances are very intense. When the baby lies in its mother's arms, it is well supported on its back by the mother's knees, with the soles of its feet against the mother's stomach. This comforting experience urges the newborn to look into its mother's eyes. Then the words that she usually addresses to the baby act as an acoustic envelope, conveying a strong emotional message, which is then completed and integrated by breast-feeding. The mother acts as binder for the integration, as long as she is able to accept her child's messages and feed them back, adding significance to them. When the relationship functions like this, integration will be promoted.

The child who rejects contact will also dislike being in the position of having its back and neck supported. Reporting the treatment of a child who used to avert his eyes and was affected by major psychopathological disorders, Madam Haag (1988) pointed out the importance of some sensory stimulus to produce the first eye contact: such as that produced by her foot touching the nape of the baby's neck when he crawled towards her. Thus Madame Haag's considerations emphasize the importance of placing the newborn child in this position for some periods during the day inside the incubator. For this purpose, the nurse's and parents' hands are used besides the hammock itself. This technique, as Fava Vizziello, Zorzi, and Bottos (1992), have emphasized, not only favours the physical containment of the little baby, but also facilitates visual perception and thus the child's attempt to seek the gaze of his parents and of the staff, beside the incubator. We started putting this technique into practice in our newborn intensive care unit about two years ago, with great benefit.

Disorders can develop not only in children affected by sensory deficiencies or injuries to the nervous system; some children have a greater need than others for their mother, to function in a way that promotes the integration of their sense organs; others seem constitutionally more able to develop this integration from within. In children who are constitutionally less able to integrate, disorders can develop if they have a mother who unconsciously colludes with these less vital aspects of the child. Whatever the roots of the pathological situation—sensory deficiency from injuries to the sense organs or nervous system, or constitutional factors—it is clear that children are visibly tormented by the paranoid and confusional anxieties that prevent them from finding a way out of their persistent auto-sensory condition.

It is usually the mother, or both parents, who may be in a position to help the child to differentiate by recognizing, accepting, and linking up the violent emotional aspects that cannot be tolerated by the child. In the observation sessions with Francesca, we can see how her relationship with her mother binds the integration: only when (as here) the mother is able to receive the baby's messages and transmit them back again with added significance will integration be promoted. The mother plays the unconscious role (reverie) of linking the various sensory factors, because she can grasp their intention and expressiveness; thus she widens the little girl's experience and supports her in her activity (Bion, 1962).

> During the session when Francesca is 3 months and 1 day old, she is ill. It is her first illness. During the first part of the session she is miserable and uncomfortable, but after a good breast-feed, listening to her mother's loving talk, the baby looks decidedly more cheerful: she stops sucking and responds to her mother's affectionate words with quite articulate and expressive sounds.

We can understand from this how it is through these sensory and emotional routes that the child discovers its own drive and willingness to integrate and learn. Therefore the first priority in the treatment of children affected by serious communication and attention disorders is to help their parents to find these routes of contact and mobilize their receptive functions. This type of consulting involves first of all describing the symptoms and alarm signals, learning to pay attention to them, and then enabling parents to respond in a way aimed at changing them. (These aspects are dealt with in greater detail in chapter seven.)

In my experience, the major types of psychopathology to which newborns in a neonatal pathology ward are exposed are psychosis, the "minimal brain dysfunction syndrome" (the "specific development disorders" in the new DSM IIIR terminology), and psychosomatic disorders. It is clearly very important to identify the distinctive symptoms of these three major areas of infant psychiatry, because only through carefully directed environmental intervention is it possible to obtain a "spectacular" remission of the disorder (to use the French authors' definition: Cramer, 1974; Haag, 1985; Houzel & Bastard, 1988; Lebovici, 1978, 1983; Male, Doumic-Girard, Benhamon, & Schott, 1975; Soulé, Houzel, & Bollaert, 1976; Stork, 1983; Watillon-Naveau, 1992).

This is a very major and widespread problem, which affects a large number of infants hospitalized in neonatal intensive care wards, especially those whose weight is less than 1.500 kg. In 1991, Volpe reported that out of 42,000 newborns below 1.550 kg who are born every year in the United States, about 85% survive. Of these, 5–15% develop cerebral palsy, but 25–50% more suffer from a "minor disorder", characterized usually by a learning deficiency. The percentage with a relational-cognitive disorder is even higher (40–64%) in newborns below 1000 g (Collin, Halsey, & Anderson, 1991; Fazzi et al., 1987). [The validity of the neuropsychological prevention model adopted within the neonatal intensive care unit of our hospital and described in this book has been confirmed during the children's follow-ups after being discharged from hospital. The frequency rate of cerebral palsy among newborns at Treviglio Hospital between 1977 and 1987 is 1.4 per thousand—lower than that reported by the Hagbergs and colleagues (B. Hagberg, 1989; B. Hagberg, & Hagberg, 1993; B. Hagberg, Hagberg, &

Olow, 1984; B. Hagberg, Hagberg, & Zatterstrom, 1989; B. Hagberg, Hagberg, Olow, & Von Wendt, 1989; G. Hagberg, 1989), by Badalamenti, Bonarrio, Canziani, & Mangano (1986), by Ellenberg and Nelson (1988), and by Trevisan et al. (1986). Evaluation between 1977 and 1987 of the case history of newborns with a birth weight less than 1.500 kg shows a 6% rate of cerebral palsy and a 19% rate of "mild to moderate" relational–cognitive disorders. The outcome for newborns of less than 1.000 kg from 1986 onwards is equally encouraging; they are more favourable than those reported by Volpe (1991a, 1991b), Fazzi et al. (1987), and Collin et al. (1991), with similar categories of children. Chapter eight explores further the psychopathological problems of children who go on to develop cerebral palsy.]

Early psychoses, or general development disorders, according to DSM III

The most frequent alarm symptoms are: gaze aversion, the absence of smiling, stiff mimicry, stereotyping, irritability, postural anomalies, and feeding and sleeping disorders.

A fairly constant symptom in newborn children who are at risk of developing a psychosis is the upsetting of their biological rhythms. The rhythmic character of these seems to be the expression of a genetic potential, of a maturation process of the nervous system, and, finally, of a multifaceted response to the environment. The alternation of light and dark is probably one of the most obvious external rhythms, but the alternation of noise and silence is similarly important, and so (according to Mills, 1975) is the attention devoted by adults to the child: this makes the relationship of adult and child a major factor in rhythm adjustment.

During the first months of life, major changes occur in the sleep–waking cycle and distribution, such as a gradual reduction of sleeping, a doubling of the active waking state, and a significant reduction in crying; these find expression in the child's increasingly more complex learning and relational abilities.

But in the case of infants at risk of incurring psychotic disorders this is not the case. Here a complete upsetting of noctodiurnal rhythms can often be observed, and a failure to undergo the gradual rhythm changes described above. The upsetting of circadian rhythms is mainly due to the onset of a state of irritability (as described in my works: Negri, 1984, 1986). This pathological condition would be suddenly manifested by the child, without any apparent external reason, thus triggering an uncontainable excitement: eye-lids are suddenly dropped, the body is shaken by a painful hyperexcitement, the head is abruptly thrown backward or forward, the hands open and close rhythmically while upper limbs bend. This state may last for a few hours and sometimes recurs frequently during the day. It is the manifestation of a deep anxiety, which isolates the newborn in its crying, so that attempts at soothing and communication by the mother are fruitless.

The upsetting of the sleep–waking rhythm can also manifest itself in excessive sleeping, especially during the day, whereas at night difficulties may lead to an actual reversal of the sleep–waking rhythm. In cases where there are no nocturnal problems, parents report that these children are "too good"— they just "sleep and eat". When they are awake, they tend to keep their head turned forward, with their eyelids semi-closed and with an "undifferentiated" look—sometimes downwards, upwards, or sideways, sometimes turned towards the contents of the room, but in an amorphous way. Their posture may also appear flaccid, suggesting suspected hypotonia. Parents describe the behaviour of these children as passive and indifferent to sounds and voices.

Starting from the second month of life, the posture of the head can be very significant. It may be kept predominantly turned forwards, as already mentioned, or it may be turned slightly backwards. These postures, which are sometimes wrongly interpreted as neurological disorders, show a lack of integration of the child's sensory functions—the look, the use of mouth and hands. In particular, the child tends to "avert its eyes", so that it manages very intelligently to elude someone's look (intelligence being, as Meltzer [Meltzer et al., 1975, p. 9] says, "a mental process which operates at great speed"). Sometimes, in order better to escape looking into people's eyes, the baby lowers his eyelids and pretends to sleep. To illustrate this we may take the case of Giuseppe, an attractive 3-month-old boy with intelligent and lively eyes. Yet, according to neighbours, it was as though he could not see—staring in front of him and averting his gaze; to his mother's annoyance people would pass their hand before his eyes to try to make him react. His mother told me she felt that instead of looking at her, he was spying on her when she was not looking: "He looks at me behind my back." It seemed that he really could not tolerate being looked in the eyes, especially at close proximity; when this happened, he would blush, drop his eye-lids, and burst out crying, as if he wanted to get rid of the experience—acting, in fact, as though he were trying to evacuate faeces.

This child had undergone a very traumatic obstetric procedure during his delivery and was consequently admitted to the neonatal intensive care unit. He seemed to enjoy being held, however, and listening to his mother's words; but he refused to allow his experiences to be put together and relocated outside himself in the presence of an object. The birth experience had been so persecutory for him that it led him to make excessive use of projection and splitting processes. It was not surprising that this baby was affected by a form of eczema on the upper surface of his foot, for in such cases psychosomatic disturbances such as eczema and colic are very frequent. These show the children's excessive tendency to expel, to isolate emotions and sensations in their body because they experience them in such persecutory terms that they cannot be ingested mentally.

Sometimes, from the very first moments of being held in their mother's arms, they have such an intense hyperkinesia of their four limbs that the arms and upper part of the body take up an attitude similar to that of boxers when fighting. This postural anomaly improves with treatment, which reveals that it was essentially a means of isolation from their environment. These children seldom smile, and if they do, their smile holds hardly any communicatory significance. Parents often report a sort of "mimic rigidity". To explain this, they usually bring the child's photograph album and show how from the very first pictures taken at birth the child has not seemed ever to change its expression while growing.

In some cases, a backward-leaning head posture may be accompanied by motor manifestations that make the child's tendency to isolate itself even clearer: thus the head is turned backwards or in the direction away from the mother's face, so as to better avoid her gaze; the upper limbs are bent, abducted, and stiffened in an attitude of "distancing", as though the child wanted to avoid all contact with the mother; or there may be a sudden, abrupt, violent arching of the trunk, as if to jerk itself away from the mother's lap. The picture is usually completed by "gaze aversion", often with protruding tongue, and may also be followed by the onset of gesture stereotypes, starting from the fourth month. There may be feeding problems as well. Giuseppe, in fact, starts sucking greedily and angrily; then he continues very slowly; his mother reports: "He seems afraid that the bottle will be taken away." Regurgitation and vomiting often occur, up to the rejection of the food itself, as in the case of a little girl examined at 4 months of age, who burst out crying desperately at the mere sight of the bottle. Passivity in feeding can also often be the case, as with Federica, whose parents reported: "Federica has never had feeding problems, but has just accepted being fed without any pleasure, any involvement; she has just let it be done as if she were a robot."

In similar situations, in which the fragmenting and splitting processes are particularly serious, the anxiety about disintegration can manifest itself through "plastic hypertonia", as it is called: children stay paralysed in their postures, frightened by the slightest change, and they enter a state of irritability. Every tiny movement makes them feel anxious; held in one's arms, they remain stiff and tense. They only relax their muscles in sleep, but their sleep is nonetheless extremely tormented.

These children are described by their parents as being "like dolls", owing to their postural rigidity; and when they start to walk, they look like marionettes, moving jerkily by fits and starts, with no suppleness or smoothness. They are not hindered in their feeding, but they eat like robots, as though they cannot make any distinction between inside and outside, between themselves and the food. Catastrophic anxieties may be unleashed by even a slight cold, as was the case with a girl examined at age 6: "It was impossible to blow her nose; it was as though she feared she would break into pieces. She still can't accept it; I have to do everything for her."

The two latter cases, if not given appropriate treatment in time, may easily turn into different forms of schizophrenic or disintegration psychoses.

The psychosomatic syndrome

The major alarm symptoms are psychosomatic phenomena, such as tremor, hiccups, irritability, motor restlessness, postural anomalies, and disorders of the skin, respiration, feeding, and sleeping.

Many authors recognize the dangerous situation underlying psychosomatic symptoms (Di Cagno & Ravetto, 1982; E. Gaddini, 1981; R. Gaddini, 1980; Harris, cited in Negri, 1973, p. 886; Kreisler, 1981; Kreisler, Fain, & Soulé, 1967; Rosenfeld, 1978; Soulé et al., 1976; Sperling, 1953; Winnicott, 1966). The ego finds itself in its very early stages faced with highly destructive and intolerable primitive phantasies, which are turned immediately and unconsciously into the psychosomatic disease.

The absolute dependence on the environment and the biological immaturity of early life leads researchers to identify several factors as causing a psychosomatic pathological situation. Winnicott (1966), in particular, dwells on the onset of the disorder; he identifies a non-integrated primary state in the newborn's early life, soon after birth. The integration process depends on the responsiveness of the mother. If the mother offers the newborn a firm reality on which to depend, then the psychosomatic integration (the "I am" state) will take place, and the psyche will live happily inside the body; but if the maternal containment (of arms, eyes, and voice) is insufficient at a time when the self is not yet organized, then maturation problems and errors in mental metabolization occur. This means that the physical ingredients of the first sensory experiences cannot be metabolized into psychical products.

From this point of view, psychosomatic disorders can be regarded as defects in integration, and they are defined by

Winnicott (1966) as "primary anxieties" leading to "a special form of splitting that takes place in the mind, but along psychosomatic lines". It is a sort of splitting that is developed in the mind to defend against the persecutors of the rejected world, which are trapped in the body; this splitting acts as a defence against highly destructive phantasies (Di Cagno & Ravetto, 1982; Rosenfeld, 1978). This aspect has led most authors (Kreisler et al., 1967; Kreisler, 1981; Pinkerton, 1965; Soulé et al., 1976; Spitz, 1951) to emphasize the mother's role at the onset of psychosomatic disorders, taking into account such things as separations or losses, a new pregnancy during the first year, or psychopathological characteristics of the mother.

Other authors regard alterations in wider models of family interaction as decisive factors in the onset of the pathology. Thus Kreisler (1981) identifies a deprivation somatic disorder, due mainly to the child's hospitalization or to a so-called "blank" relationship with a mother who is not able to be emotionally involved with her child. In addition to this, he describes a somatic disorder induced by hyperstimulation or excessive excitement, which results in some of the most common functional disorders such as colic, sleeping problems, or laryngospasms. Continuous excitement directed by parents onto a given functional sphere (feeding or evacuation) engenders disorders such as anorexia, constipation, or irritable colon. Furthermore, Kreisler (1981) detects a type of hyperstimulation in overprotective maternal attitudes, excluding the father, which can lead to a symbiotic relationship detrimental to the achievement of the separation–individuation process.

In the seriously preterm newborn, the conditions of both deprivation and hyperstimulation will be found, alternating with one another. Therefore there is an increased risk of the onset of the above-mentioned disorders related to claustrophobic anxieties.

Many authors mention genetic factors when they refer to the child's "psychosomatic constitution". This is a concept that has different interpretations. There is a wide-ranging individual variability among newborns in heart-rate, skin temperature, and responses of the autonomic nervous system. Great flexibility is required on the part of the mother to respond to these individual needs. Pinkerton (1965) describes different types of

children: strong or weak, with sensitive and vulnerable personalities, as well as children "allergic to emotional stresses". Most
authors have stressed the particularly hypertonic behaviour of
children who develop colic during the first three months.
Kreisler (1981) refers to "vulnerable personalities", whose behavioural structure may be a suitable ground for a somatic
disorder. Yet, as Kreisler stresses, this is a psychic structure
that operates for the time being, not an unchangeable organization, since in the child nothing becomes defined until adolescence.

The above considerations underline the complexity of the
"psychophysical" condition of the child, from birth and during
its first year of life in particular. During this period, the drama
of what Schneider (1968) defines as the "psychosomatic fact" (a
situation whose biological aspect is inseparable from its psychological one) is lived out.

This distinctive feature of the newborn—the fusion of
psyche and soma—highlights a problem in terminology. Is it,
then, possible to talk about illness, or is it better to refer to
symptoms or even to a different mode of organization or of non-
organization, according to the various stages in the child's
development?

On the one hand, the progressive perspective implicit in
development tends to override the distinction between symptoms and disease; on the other hand, a detailed description of
defence mechanisms justifies making a distinction. The fact
that at this age, in my experience, the illness is always associated with a whole series of symptoms suggests a suitable
definition to be "the psychophysical syndrome" (as suggested
by Greenacre, 1958) or, more simply, "the psychosomatic syndrome" (Negri, 1989c). This term is wide and not too rigid in its
implications, respecting the development context and abstain-
ing from a predictive assessment.

This clarification is important because, especially with
young children, it is essential to distinguish the symptoms
from the disease. The younger the child, the more will psychosomatic symptoms be used for communication, to find a way of
facing and understanding the problem. As an example of this I
may take the case of Simone, whom I followed personally within
the framework of infant observation from his birth until the age

of five. At 2½ he had to cope with the birth of a sister and with starting nursery school; he had frequent and prolonged episodes of bronchitis, colds, and flu, despite having a strong physical constitution. At this stage in his development, Simone came across so many serious emotional problems that he needed to resort to physical illness to express them all. At a time like this it is important for the child's message to be understood by those caring for him, to help him to tolerate and work through these deeply conflictual feelings, a necessary stage in his development. But the emotional situation of a child affected by a psychosomatic disorder or syndrome is, of course, much more complex and serious.

In children less than a year old, the pathology can manifest itself as eczema, colic, merycism (ruminative regurgitation), asthma, or gastrointestinal or other disorders. It is always associated with other somatic disturbances, such as affective spasms, tremor, hypertonia, sleeping and feeding disorders, etc.—indeed, the whole range of symptoms. In these circumstances, parents usually express their worry about two aspects of the child, one being expressed in physical terms and related to the newborn's initial non-integration, and the other more specifically concerning features of omnipotence that they have observed in the child's behaviour.

The first, physical, aspect includes such things as atopic dermatitis, asthma, affective spasms, tremor, hiccups, irritability, the head held exaggeratedly backwards or forwards, hypertonia, hypermotility, vomiting, colic, digestive and sleeping disorders. The second aspect, of omnipotence, includes the following characteristics: withdrawing from being cuddled, merycism, self-feeding, impatience at being kept waiting, accusatory looks, constantly calling people's attention to them, being "cunning, crafty, false, reckless, obstinate, slow-witted, ambitious, arrogant, demanding" (these are parents' expressions.

The omnipotent control is a defence mechanism triggered by anxieties related to the failure in integration. Usually it greatly hurts parents, and from a psychodynamic point of view it manifests "the child's exasperated need to possess its mother, to enter inside her and finally control and manipulate her from within, shutting out all other experiences" (Harris, cited in Negri, 1973, p. 886). This explains the enormous separation difficulties encountered by these children, as well as their tyrannical and possessive attitude, their destructiveness, and their anxieties about death and illness, which emerge in their behaviour and play once they become older and are brought to consultation.

From the psychodynamic point of view, there are strong similarities between the psychosomatic disorder and the minimal brain damage syndrome. In both disorders, the capacity for symbolization is not well developed, and the depressive component is predominant.

When analysing psychosomatic disorders in the newborn, one must not forget that the psychosomatic pattern development takes place within a specific mother–child, parent–child relation. In particular, there may emerge the mother's need to maintain the child's dependence. Even though she may often complain about the burden of her child's illness, she may be able to give love and care only to an ill child. This will cast a sort of magic spell on the child, reassuring him that he will never have to suffer from the loss of his mother: thus he becomes dependent on her.

The child's collusion with the mother's unconscious needs may lead to feelings of guilt in the mother, thus producing an unconscious denial of the illness, as well as an apparent rejection of her child. These women are faced with an unsolved dependency problem, which fuels phantasies of omnipotence. If the unconscious attitude of the mother is not taken into consideration, the treatment is bound to fail; she will feel unable to return for consultation and the child's condition will worsen.

* * *

I would now like to report some findings derived from the case histories of 58 children affected by the "psychosomatic syndrome", who were first examined at between 2 and 3 months of age. These same children were then followed at the paediatric clinic, in the department devoted to newborns at risk.

As already mentioned, the illness affecting the young patient is always accompanied by a whole series of symptoms. There were, for example, 1 case of merycism, 9 cases of colic, and 23 cases of cradle cap; feeding, digestive, and vomiting problems were noted in 25 children; 43% of all cases were affected by major sleeping disorders. The illness has its roots in the very early stages of development, as seems confirmed by the fact that 79% presented major problems even during pregnancy or delivery (threatened abortions, dystocias).

Sometimes a deeply depressive element in the personality of the mother emerges from the case history. As Palacio Espasa and Manzano (1982) point out, an incompletely resolved mourning experience can always be identified in the histories of these women. The child with its symptoms embodies an aspect of the psychic situation of the mother who is still affected by unsolved separation problems. Giannotti, Lanza, and Del Pidio (1984), in particular, attach great importance to the parents' unconscious phantasies as the substratum of the child's phantasy world. Already in the womb, the child seems to be influenced by the pathobiological model of the parental couple, especially of the mother. The more pathological the model, the more difficulty the child will have in the differentiation and integration of its mental and bodily functioning. He will then re-enact phenomena that belong in the parents' relationship, precisely according to the quantity and quality of the unconscious phantasies projected onto him. Giannotti thus refers to a primary trauma, which seems to have affected the child already *in utero*, influencing the normal syntonic coordination and interaction between a certain organ or systems and the rest of the body.

The "minimal brain dysfunction syndrome"

Specific development disorders, according to the DSM IIIR

The most frequent alarm symptoms are: slipping away of eye-contact, motor restlessness, and postural anomalies.

The M.B.D. syndrome is a clinical picture that is frequently found in the English research literature. In Italy it has been explored in particular by Benedetti, Curatolo, and Galletti (1978), De Negri (1990), and Guareschi-Cazzullo (1980, 1991).

Its problems of diagnosis, care, and treatment are still unsolved. It concerns the so-called "minor pathologies" of infancy, not including autism and cerebral palsy.

In children affected by M.B.D., movement abnormalities and psychological difficulties coexist, yet without resulting in serious impairment, as in autism or cerebral palsy. Instead, there is a clumsiness of movement, difficulty in coordination, hyperkinesia, or hypokinesia; psychic disorders exist at the same time, but they are less severe than in autism. Overall mental retardation is minimal: the child manifests an attention deficit, inadequate social adjustment, emotional instability, impulsiveness, and intolerance of frustration. Many pathological symptoms have been described, to be included within the definition of the syndrome. Some ten symptoms have been identified as distinctive elements of this pathological picture—(1) hyperactivity (the hyperkinetic syndrome); (2) motor perceptual impairments; (3) emotional instability; (4) overall co-ordination impairment; (5) attention disorders; (6) impulsiveness; (7) memory and thinking disorders; (8) specific learning impairments (writing, reading, arithmetic, etc.); (9) language and hearing disorders; (10) doubtful neurological signs and electro-encephalographic irregularities (Clements, 1966). The major symptoms concern attention deficit and learning difficulties (reading, writing, calculation). These problems are accompanied by a marked psychomotor instability or motor deficiencies such as those already pointed out: a lack of coordination and awkwardness of movement; hypokinesia; dyspraxias and dyspractognosies.

Along with the language and speech disorders, dyspraxias, and other specific learning impairments, "hyperkinesia" has for some time (since 1967) been recognized as a special syndrome. Its features are distractibility, short attention span, impulsiveness, aggressiveness, mood fluctuations, and, finally, the peculiar response to amphetamines it entails. The hyperkinetic syndrome used to be regarded simply as a descriptive category, owing to the uncertainty of its neuro-and psychopathological structure and to doubt about its being able to maintain its distinctiveness in the long term as a clinical manifestation. In fact, however, it has passed the time test and is now regarded as a diagnostic category included in the II axis of DSM IIIR, where it is defined as "attention deficit disturbance with hyper-activity" (D.D.A.I.).

The clinical picture of the specific development disorders, even those concerning a minor pathology, leads to a chain of disorders that intensify with time, resulting in major social and school adjustment problems for the child (Hadders-Algra, Touwen, Olinga, & Huisjés, 1985). Impairments are usually detected very late, at school age, owing to difficulties in learning and emotional adjustment, in spite of the fact that neuro-paediatricians have long since shown the correlation between the temporary anomalies ("soft signs") and the minimal brain damage syndrome.

Amiel-Tison and colleagues (Amiel-Tison & Grenier, 1980; Amiel-Tison & Dube, 1985) define as temporary disorders those phenomena which appear, respectively, during the first, second, and third quarters of the first year of life but are no longer found at the age of 1. During the first quarter, a hyperexciteability and hypertonia can be observed in the upper part of the body; in the second and third quarters, there is a persistence of the primitive reflexes, a failure of the passive tone in the lower limbs to relax, and axial tone anomalies with failure of the sitting position and persistent overall straighten-ing out, in addition to hyperexcitability. These anomalies are temporary phenomena, because at the age of 1 there is no visible difference between these children and those who have developed normally. Yet, according to Amiel-Tison and col-leagues, this is only an "apparent return to normality" and is part of a certain stage of development. The damage becomes temporarily silent but will emerge in various ways over the following years, in the form of behaviour disorders, fine motility anomalies, and learning deficiencies. These authors highlight the significance of a fact that is already generally known: namely, that although there is a substantial reduction of the risk of major brain injury thanks to the present highly ad-vanced intervention procedures on newborns, specialists are, instead, being confronted with alarming percentages of the so-called "late" minor pathologies in infants.

In 1972, for example, in a case record of 300 newborns weighing 2000 gr or less, Drillien described a syndrome of "transient dystonia". At 2 and 3 years of age, children who had previously been dystonic were much more likely to have mental impairment and hyperactive behaviour than those children of similar birthweights who had not exhibited abnormal neurologic signs.

In considering the link between temporary neurological anomalies and learning difficulties at school age, Amiel-Tison and colleagues distinguish between an organic aspect on the one hand and, on the other, the cause–effect relation with a perinatal disorder. This calls into question the nature of the "minimal brain dysfunction" (M.B.D.), which assumes the existence of minor injuries of the white substance that would show only temporarily at an initial stage of development. Cortical lesions, however, would emerge only later and would affect the long-term prognosis. Nevertheless, these anatomical and clinical assumptions are not confirmed by tomodensitometry.

In a case record by Bergstrom and Bille (1978) of 46 children between the ages of 14 and 15, who had been diagnosed as having M.B.D., only 15 (32%) showed signs of encephelatrophy or other forms of atrophy. Bergstrom, Bille, and Rasmussen (1984) considered a case record of 89 boys and 20 girls with minor neurodevelopmental disorders, and 25% showed aberrations on CT (computed tomography) scans. The incidence of manifest left-handedness and of developmental language disorders was not higher among children with pathological CT findings than among those with normal ones. It is well known that in infant neuropsychiatry there is not a precise correlation between damage to the brain and also extremely severe disorders such as cerebral palsy or the psychoses. The fact is, a careful examination of the literature makes it clear how far we are from establishing whether or not the minimal brain dysfunction's etiopathogenesis derives from neuropathological or psychopathological aspects, or to what extent both aspects are implicated.

Already in 1962, in his paper on "Minimal Chronic Brain Syndromes in Children", Richmon S. Paine pointed out the multiplicity of etiologic factors involved, referring to the high percentage of preterm newborns in the case-record by Knobloch and Pasaminick (1959) and of children with a family history of mental disorders in Mautner's (1959) case-record. He also stressed the prevailing presence of severe emotional and behavioural problems. He regretted the fact that psychiatrists are reluctant to prescribe psychotherapy to children affected by disorders whose "organic origin" was suspect. Paine, therefore, prescribes for M.B.D. cases treatment aimed at improving the relationship situations of the child.

Likewise, Paul H. Wender (1971) considers the same clinical picture from more than one perspective. His interpretation of the minimal brain damage syndrome is very broad. When considering the etiopathological aspect, he points out several factors of a hereditary, organic, and psychogenetic character. When considering the clinical picture, he does not rule out as possible M.B.D. subcategories the neurotic, psychopathic, and schizophrenic syndromes, nor the "hyperactive syndrome and specific learning impairment". He stresses the importance of psychological problems, and in evaluating the efficacy of drugs, he seems to prefer amphetamines, stating that "Drugs can help the child learn reading, acting on its attention, but they can improve neither its understanding of the text nor its learning skills. They may quieten the child, thus making it more susceptible to being more easily accepted by the environment, but they cannot convey to it the experience of having been favourably welcome in the past." Wender also assumes that depressive features are at the basis of the M.B.D. symptomatology, and that the favourable response to tricyclic antidepressant drugs seems to confirm this assumption—hence, he points out, the need to combine the drug therapy with psychological treatment.

Through the analysis of a case history of 462 preterm newborns, examined from 1958 until 1969, Lezine (1977), in collaboration with Berges, identified the "late syndrome of the preterm infant" in children between 3 and 10 years of age, who were affected by school difficulties and problems of social adjustment. This syndrome is characterized by a disturbance of practognostic functions, by a failure to maintain an integrated body image, and by emotional and relational disorders.

Although the authors seem to abstain from making any interpretation of their findings—so that their work is entitled simply "Syndrome"—Lezine (1977) herself explicitly wonders what hypotheses about injury could be formulated that would explain the above disorders. She recognizes that most authors include the psychopathology of newborns at risk in the M.B.D.

framework because it is assumed that these children may have suffered brain injuries during pregnancy or delivery. But with reference to the broader scope of the case histories, the author also points out that the neurological disorders that were identified or suspected at birth do not seem to have any predictive value, at least as far as the development of the practognostic functions is concerned. She also stresses that the neurological disorders identified during the first few days of life can be aggravated by unfavourable environmental factors, such as insufficient stimulation, or the child being prevented from establishing bonds of affection with the people surrounding it (Negri, 1985).

Kreisler (Kreisler & Soulé, 1985) also highlights the relational problem as well as the somatic fragility when considering the principal features of psychopathology in the preterm newborn. He identifies early disorders in which some irregularities appear during the first two years of life. When these are sufficiently serious, they may lead to diagnoses closer to psychosis. In the so-called "late" disorders (appearing from 2 to 3 years until later school age), Kreisler outlines the onset of the syndrome as already described by Berges (Berges, Lezine, Harrison, & Boisselier, 1969); he also considers a picture (defined as the most extreme form of the Berges syndrome) in which intelligent children have such severe disturbances in their learning and identity, that they enter the diagnostic category of psychosis.

Kreisler and Soulé (1985), like Lezine (1977), call attention to the early life conditions of the newborn at risk, in order to understand the psychopathological aspects better: "not because they specifically refer to this condition, but because they affect these children with alarmingly high rates". The same conclusions are drawn by Moceri and Pagnin (1983) in their clinical assessment of 62 newborns: all were born prematurely, spent a certain length of time in the incubator, and were brought for consultation at between 4 and 11 years of age, owing to behavioural difficulties.

The psychopathological problems of these children, which emerge during school age in a particularly alarming way, can only be understood if the importance of the maternal function—defined by Bick as the "skin"—is taken into account. Bick

(1968) points out that in the initial state of non-integration, the newborn feels the need for an object that can show it is able to hold together the different parts of its personality. Ideally, this object would be represented by the nipple in its mouth, by the mother's way of holding it and speaking, and by her familiar smell: a complete picture to meet its sensual needs. The containing object is experienced by the newborn on a mental level as a skin, bounding the limits of the internal space in which thinking takes shape.

A defective development of the primary functions of the "skin" can derive from maternal insufficiency and from phantasies damaging an integrated and then integrating introjection.

This insufficient containment is experienced by the child as a dangerous situation, resulting in parts of the self being spilled out and excluded; it becomes a source of extremely primitive fragmentation anxieties, which lead the child to build up a "second skin" as a sort of defence around itself. When this happens, the supportive function of a true internal object is replaced by a fragile muscular independence, both mental and physical, as a result of omnipotently taking over the sensory and mental equipment needed for the containing function. All this can lead to the development of a two-dimensional personality in which the identification with the object is adhesive, superficial, shallow, with no concept of space or time. It is founded on the imitation of superficial qualities, rather than on learning from experience through processes of projection and introjection.

The concept of the two-dimensional personality clearly illuminates the psychodynamic situation of the child with learning impairments or, more generally, of the child affected by M.B.D., whose main feature is a failure in containment, which prevents the establishment of an internal space where thinking can take place. The defence against primitive anxieties about disintegration is expressed through muscular and oral activities, which replace the "skin" function. Thus the significance becomes clear of the hyperkinesias, rhythmical activities, ritualized compulsions, behavioural disorders, and psychomotor instability described by Kreisler (Kreisler & Soulé, 1985) in the context of early infancy: "I could often observe in children who had been born prematurely some tics or even more frequently, forms of instability. . . . What struck me most in these children was the absence of symbolization and of mental working out."

If one bears in mind, therefore, the "fragmentation anxieties" to which the newborn is exposed when in an intensive care unit, it becomes possible to understand the meaning of the "soft signs" (as described by British authors), or of the "temporary anomalies" (as described by French authors), as well as what I have defined as "alarm symptoms"—tremor, hiccups, sneezing, psychosomatic manifestations. All these are expressions of the newborn's containment difficulties, whereas the distal hypertonia and the motor restlessness are mechanisms of defence, employed in the face of a dangerous situation.

"Distal hypertonia" manifests itself during the neurological assessment and appears spontaneously during the day, especially when the child is undressed or bathed, or when it is in any new or different situation. I have defined "motor restlessness"—Drillien's (1972) minor dystonia—in other research works as an intensification of the spontaneous motility that can be detected soon after birth. It is associated with an intolerance of eye-contact with the mother or parents, which likewise illustrates the child's special difficulty with the relationship. The fleeting gaze does not usually refer only to the relational aspect, but more generally to the child's way of looking at people or objects in the room, thus manifesting a very early major attention deficit. This is usually followed by a peculiar attitude when being held in someone's arms: the child often demands to be held, but he wants to do it his own way, without ever relaxing or clinging to his parent's body and accepting dependency; instead, he wriggles and tosses about, always maintaining a rather tense muscular tone, or remaining quite isolated in himself, despite the bodily contact. With time, the picture can turn into a true hyperkinesia: the child moves relentlessly from one position to the next, never stopping, apart from a few seconds spent in fidgeting with one object after another. This attitude becomes even more evident in behaviour when the child starts walking—which occurs quite early—showing a marked motor instability.

Psychomotor instability in the child is often associated with rather destructive, poorly integrated, and un-symbolic play activity. Other features are also reported by parents. In addition to "nervousness" and difficulty in relaxing and being cuddled when held, parents also report a markedly self-sufficient attitude in the child. This becomes apparent from the very beginning: "He wants to get the bottle and feed himself; he looks at me evasively, as though he really disliked me. . . . I'm frightened by the way he grabs things, by his animated manner; I am afraid he may become too reckless when he grows up." Already at this very early stage of development, an intolerance of frustration emerges. These children cannot wait for their bottle; they want everything immediately.

The above observations show the omnipotent attitudes that, together with the marked muscular activity, determine the development of what Esther Bick (1968) has described as the "second skin". This is responsible for the two-dimensional character of the personalities of these children and for the adhesiveness underlying their severe learning impairments.

It is, however, possible to detect this condition very early, owing to the semiological features listed above; and with the help of adequate and appropriate modification of the child's environment, it is possible to change the child's outlook and attitude to relationships and to obtain a satisfactory improvement in terms of a more balanced personality development.

CHAPTER SEVEN

Treatment

The post-discharge follow-up of the newborn at risk has a therapeutic significance, and so the methodology employed there is similar to that adopted in cases requiring actual treatment. In these cases, changes are introduced in response to the clinical picture (as illustrated in greater detail below). During the examination it is very important to think about the degree of weakening of the life instinct which all newborns at risk undergo, both on account of possible brain damage and because of the traumatic therapeutic procedures. It must also be borne in mind that the newborn tends to believe that these seriously persecutory situations originate in the mother. Given its specific mental apparatus, it is in fact very perceptive of its mother's anxiety, which, especially at the beginning, hinders the adequacy of her response to the child's complex communications (Salzberg-Wittenberg, 1990). Therefore the mother's anxiety is experienced by the child as extremely threatening and imminent, and this aggravates the child's emotional difficulties.

This situation has often been confirmed during my work and experience of prevention techniques. A discouraged mother once said to me, of her baby: "He really seems to dislike me!" Indeed, many children, especially those most seriously affected, seem to prefer their fathers. Awareness of this problem and of the defence dynamics deriving from it was an important factor in initiating prevention techniques with preterm newborns from the first moments of their hospitalization (as described in chapter three). It also helps us to understand the deeply depressive situation faced by parents—by mothers in particular—immediately after the child's discharge from hospital.

As Martha Harris (1966) writes:

> It is important that the parents come together, jointly responsible for their child, and that they are enabled to express their problem, their feelings of helplessness as parents, to an "expert" who is supposed to have some experience in dealing with these problems. But not an expert who, from the height of superior knowledge, treats them as helpless children, instructing them in what to do, or in what they should not have done, thereby confirming their own childish fears of being discovered to be inadequate and fraudulent parents incapable of responsibility and dependent therefore upon some higher authority. The helpful expert in such a situation is one who can have a role analogous to that of the understanding mother with the distressed baby, who receives the projection of the infant's anxiety, is with it, and enables it to cope better with pain because it no longer feels alone. A child who does not thrive and respond to the mother's efforts to alleviate his distress, evokes all her own infantile helplessness and loneliness. Such a mother can easily lose touch with the experience that she has acquired, and lose faith in the defence she has built up against her inadequacy.
>
> It seems to me that I come through to the parents as someone who is in them both and in their child, and also as someone who has no magical expertise which would solve their problems for them, but who gives them the hope that talking together and attempting to understand would help in time. This encourages them to go on working upon the problem, to draw upon their own observations and intuitions, their unique knowledge of themselves and of the child, in order to find new methods of coping.

Thus a complex field of relationships can exist in consultations. As Dina Vallino Macciò (1992) writes in one of her recent important works, it is essential for the therapist to set up a "work group" with the child's parents, giving them equal responsibility. Together, the therapist and the couple work towards the objective of better understanding what is happening to the child.

My presence as a person who is receptive to the emotional atmosphere conveyed by the parents and their child, a person who thinks and tries to understand what happens during the consultation without judging or acting, therefore encourages the parents' own thinking activity and helps them to overcome the effect of disturbing behaviour in the child. In this way parents become able to observe their child closely and also find the courage to report their findings aloud, so attaching significance to their intuitions. Meanwhile, during the consultation, the child senses the change in its parents' attitude and responds to my twofold function of stimulating the parents' emotional contact and generally creating a more favourable atmosphere in the consulting room for listening and understanding. This helps the child to relax its defences and allows its parents to understand the uneasy situation better.

It is clear, considering all these aspects, that the intervention of the specialist is a particularly delicate and significant moment. Disorders of the perceptive functions, vegetative system, conditions of irritability, and motor problems all need to be taken equally into account, with a special emphasis on the symptom that seems most to affect the relationship between child and parents.

Once the child's main problem has been identified, the right words must be found to describe it to parents—to the mother in particular. This is a crucial point, because the mother may feel less frightened when she realizes that it is in fact possible to talk about aspects of her relationship with her child that have hitherto been unclear, owing to being linked with emotions so painful that they have been denied. It is an important moment, because "when parents take their small child to the observation session, they always ask for the means to better understand their child's thought mechanisms and symbol formation, so as to make it feel less lonely when coping with its difficulties"

(Vallino Macciò, 1984). The treatment intervention, therefore, serves as a bridge between parents and child, to re-establish the blocked communication; it is intended as a means of helping parents, in particular the mother, to develop more freely and happily what Bion calls the function of "reverie". This function is essential to the healthy mental development of the newborn; its repair, after being lost or impaired in the case of a child affected by a whole series of difficulties in integration of the self, is the most important and effective achievement for the child's recovery.

If the parents' state of mind is given due consideration, it becomes clear that it will not be sufficient simply to illustrate for them the dynamics underlying the reported difficulties in the consultation. What is absolutely essential, however, as Vallino Macciò (1984) points out, is to stress the most vital and positive aspects of the child as they emerge during the observation session, and to give them their full significance: "If difficulties are taken into account together with the child's resources, its suffering will be alleviated and its integration skills increased." In this way the child's integration is facilitated, and the discouraged or worried parents come to understand aspects of their child that are not easily explicable: they will not be misled, either by too close an empathic identification with their child, or by "too many details reminiscent of disaster".

Martha Harris (1980) writes:

> In these cases, the parents who are concerned about the child's fixations need to be continuously encouraged and supported in order to enable their child to develop according to its own pace, its abilities, to have the necessary time to find its spontaneous development rhythm, whereas under the pressure of their anxiety, they would be tempted to prematurely train their child to take on attitudes which would be suited to other children of the same age. [p. 125]

Meltzer (1980) adds that

> without the support of external supervision, these solicitous and thoughtful parents could easily push the child towards a bidimensional development, an adhesive identification—to imitate this and do that, to look at this or that. Our intervention therefore is mainly intended to avoid all

this. The bidimensional character can be substantially re-inforced by the collusion of parents. Especially with children affected by brain disorders or by retardation or slow development problems, the parents' anxiety for their child's social adjustment can push them to strengthen the child's tendency towards adhesive identification and the imitation of attitudes regarded as normal. [p. 125]

For this reason, longer and more frequent consultations (as suggested by Palacio Espasa & Manzano, 1982) lasting an hour and fifteen minutes are organized for the treatment of situations that, from a psychopathological point of view, are very delicate. In the standard follow-up procedure for newborns at high risk, the intervention is focused mainly on the child. However, in the case of those with serious affective disorders or severe neurological impairments, treatment aims also to take into account the projections of parents which may affect the child and further hinder its separation processes. This work requires a great deal of time and can take place only when the therapist–parent relationship has been consolidated, founded on a deep knowledge and characterized by positive feelings.

The technique used during these interventions, though not necessarily an interpretative one, enables parents to make use of the positive aspects that emerge from the transference situation with the therapist and thus to gain a deeper awareness of the problem. This can help both parents and children to overcome the parasitism within their relationship that is preventing the various individuation processes from taking place.

As an example of this, I would like to describe Giovanna, a 6-month-old girl at risk of psychosis. She was brought to me for observation by her mother, a paediatrician, who reported that she was "hypotonic and does not want to play; she is rebellious, and likes to sleep to avoid doing things". The child had already undergone many specialist examinations, such as ocular and audiometric tests, EEG, CAT scan, etc. During the first observation, although she looked around in a lively way, Giovanna showed marked relational problems, with gestural and mouth stereotypes and never looking into people's eyes but "always above", as her mother said. During the second meeting, the mother (who always came alone with her child, although her husband—an engineer, whom I met only once—seemed to be very affectionate and solicitous) overtly asked me: "Is she an autistic child?" and then burst out crying. She told me she had first become afraid when she was pregnant, after examining an autistic boy in a school where she worked as a paediatrician; she immediately feared that her forthcoming child might be like this, and she could no longer go back to that school. She had not planned to have Giovanna. She already had a 4-year-old daughter, Donatella, who, she felt, greatly needed her attention. From the beginning of her second pregnancy she had worried that a new child would cruelly deprive Donatella of her loving care, so she tried to pay special attention to her after Giovanna's birth, even allowing Donatella to suck at her breast whenever she wished. For the first three months of her life, Giovanna had been "so quiet during the day that I was happy about it".

This mother found it very difficult to relate to such a barely responsive, lazy, slow child who was yet so naughty, complaining, and stubborn, especially at night. She gave the treatment her full commitment and was very solicitous and punctual for sessions. The first period proved difficult for both of us. It was not always easy for me to contain her anxiety, in its intolerance of her little girl's slowness. Yet things gradually changed; the mother became more serene, and she seemed to become more aware of Giovanna's significant progress and of her increasing attempts to enter into contact with her mother, with me, and with the toys in the room.

The woman demonstrated clearly that she was using the treatment for herself (thus explaining her husband's absence) when she told me that she liked the area in which the hospital was situated and would have liked to live here. I also realized that she was afraid of asking for too much from me, that I might not have sufficient resources to meet her needs, when one day she sweetly told Giovanna while bottle-feeding her: "You know, if we go on eating here at the doctor's, she might get tired of us." During sessions, when the child fell asleep, she began to talk increasingly more about herself, her life, and the still unresolved problem of her reaction to the birth of her brother: "It was a real shock for me!" She still considered that event as a real injustice, describing her brother as a greedy, selfish, and arrogant person, and how she did not want Donatella to suffer as she had done. As a child, the woman had actually tried to kill her newborn brother by suffocating him. Because of this, she had been sent away from home for a while, to stay with a neighbour who loved her and looked after her well. She expressed the wish that Giovanna might become independent and sit up by herself as soon as possible, so that she would not have to neglect her elder daughter.

Soon after Giovanna's birth, Donatella had seemed to be very annoyed and troubled by her little sister's presence, especially by her reversed sleep–waking cycle. It seemed necessary to send her away from home for more than a month, to stay with a paternal aunt. In reality, it was the mother who was exhausted and irritated by the newborn's waking at night. From the point of view of the therapy, this was a very important moment—providing the evidence through which I could finally bring her to face the problems of her own confusion due to projections and identifications, which had prevented her from finding the appropriate mental space for accepting the birth of her second child. Now she will consider the possibility of needing to have some individual therapy for herself. It cannot be ruled out that Giovanna also, despite her impressive progress, may have to undergo psychotherapy eventually; early treatment is not always sufficient to fully resolve problems of psychosis.

Yet already at the age of 1, it is possible to envisage the nature of the child's future development. By this age, for example, Giuseppe (the 3-month-old child with the elusive look, mentioned in chapter six) had overcome his developmental block. He is now a beautiful 2-year-old boy, perfectly integrated, and with a very rich vocabulary. As his mother reports, he has a will of his own and knows very much what he wants, but he can also be very tender, passionate, and intelligent.

Similar progress has taken place with other children. In other cases improvement has been less definite, and not only in terms of the response and personality of the parents (although this clearly substantially influences the prognosis). Then it is recommended that individual therapy be given to the child and, usually before the age of 2, the child is referred to a psychoanalyst for observation to decide when the analysis should begin. The analyst will always remain in touch with our department. Usually parents prefer to continue consultations with me as well, although these take place less frequently. They generally like to bring the child with them and are very eager for confirmation of the improvement in their child's condition and of its ability to make use of psychotherapy and the other environmental aids provided for its benefit.

Treatment of the child affected by the *psychosomatic syndrome* is very complex. It is important to bear in mind the psychodynamics of the situation in which the child develops a physical illness and an omnipotent control of his object, as a defence against the threatening pressure of seriously destructive parts of the personality. In treatment, the environment is of fundamental importance in helping the child sort out the positive and negative aspects of its personality, so that it can tolerate the anxiety related to its destructive part, which would otherwise loom like a dangerous monster.

The success of the intervention depends not so much on the type of clinical symptomatology, as on the personality structure of the mother or parents, and the psychosomatic disorder must be considered within the context of the individual parent–child relationship. Special importance attaches to the kind of relationships established both between mother and child and between parents and therapist. The best results are obtained in cases when the mothers, despite their anxiety and fragility, have not built up any defences and are open and ready to understand their child's situation.

When I asked the mother of Michela how she managed to solve the problem of merycism, she answered: "I believed what you said, and so I told her: 'why do you put your hand in your mouth after eating? It will make all the food come up, then you'll feel bad and you'll think your mummy will feel bad too.'" I think that this situation developed favourably also because the mother understood that she could prevent her child going through the distressing process of being hung from her legs downwards, as if she were a rabbit. Michela is now 2 years old; she has overcome her problems of adjustment; the tremor that accompanied any change of posture has disappeared, as has the phobia about soft toy animals. She has progressed well, I believe, because this model for intervention is oriented not only towards the mother—who is directly involved in it—but also towards the father. There are situations in which the father's role in facilitating the separation process can be decisive, if the child's level of tolerance of frustration at that specific time is identified. This enables dramatic emotional manifestations to be received more calmly and to be given less prominence, so that greater attention can be devoted to the real needs of the child. Feelings of guilt are reduced, because there is more space for reflection.

As already mentioned, the kind of transference that is established between the mother and the therapist is very important. Whenever the child develops favourably, parents regard me as a positive figure—someone to depend on. Usually, here, the solution of the psychosomatic disorder occurs between the 8th and 10th months, after four or five consultations. But in the case of seriously depressed mothers, in whom denial, splitting, and projection mechanisms are very strong, many more difficulties are encountered, and here it is very useful to work in close cooperation with the paediatrician.

These mothers are initially very surprised and annoyed by all the questions about the psychosomatic disorder, and they soon make it clear that the child is already being followed by a paediatrician on that account. Their attitude corresponds to that described by Winnicott in relation to psychosomatic patients: not only do they split their medical care into two parts, but they fragment it even further, into many little bits, so that we, as doctors, are obliged to play only one of these tiny roles. For this reason, it is important to be very tactful and cautious with these mothers and to avoid any kind of judgement or assessment—although even so the intervention is experienced in a very persecutory way. I try to explain the child's personality characteristics very clearly, but without hiding the fact that the illness is regarded as psychosomatic, and that our words and behaviour are the only ways through which the child can give a name and identity to its own emotions, which, in turn, can facilitate its thought development, integration, and remission from the symptom.

In all these cases it is important to offer the mother the opportunity to attend more frequent and regular individual sessions, in which she can freely talk about herself and express her anxieties. This treatment would then be undertaken by one of the members of the work group, and I offer it once a confidential relationship has been established with the mother and child—usually after four or five consultations devoted to the child.

The stuttering mother of Aurora—a very beautiful and intelligent 10-month-old girl affected by eczema on her cheeks—reported that 15 days earlier the child had had a cold, and she had been afraid she would suffocate. At that time eczema had also appeared on her forehead, and she wanted to be held in her mother's arms all the time and also wanted her father to stay near and play with her. Later the mother explained: "I am always afraid she might suffocate. I sometimes dream that a necklace is suffocating her." The father added: "My wife is always so anxious . . . she's like that." By the next consultation two months later, the eczema had disappeared, and we all stressed the very satisfactory psychophysical condition of the child. The mother first mentioned the necklace dream, then some television programmes about autism, and she asked whether Aurora might develop such a serious illness. On being reassured, she asked anxiously whether the girl might eventually be affected by dyslexia.

At this point—it was the fourth consultation, and both parents had always accompanied the little girl—I felt it was the right moment to suggest further sessions specifically for the mother, in order to analyse her own anxieties rather than observing the child. The father seemed reluctant, saying: "Please forgive her, it's her character!" Yet the mother enthusiastically accepted the invitation. She has never missed a session. At present, Aurora continues to make substantial progress, perhaps helped by spending much of the day happily at her grandmother's house, while her mother—agreeing with our advice—has gone back to work again.

To take another example, Sonia—the second child of a deeply depressed mother—has also substantially improved. When she was 4 months old, she suffered from cradle cap and colic and a worrying tendency towards withdrawal. In this case, the weekly meetings with the mother were led by the physiotherapist, who was already known to the mother, as she had been referred to her 15 days after her child's birth, owing to mild neurological problems. In cases where the mother's psychopathology is more evident, therapeutic success has been achieved when the mother has been able to establish a positive transference with me: this is the kind of situation described by Palacio Espasa and Manzano (1982) as being "at the borderline of indication for short-term therapy".

Indeed, out of 52 cases of infants suffering from psychosomatic symptoms (mentioned in chapter six), 7 cases treated in the above manner did not benefit from it adequately and required specific psychoanalytic therapy—in 3 cases for the mother, and in 4 cases for the child. Regarding another 3 children from this case record, I realized that the clinical situation could not be solved simply by analysing the mother–child relationship, since there were also violent destructive aspects related strictly to the personality structure of the child. These were Riccardo, Daniele, and Elisa—all intelligent, healthy, beautiful children, 2 or 3 years old. In spite of the environmental intervention, they still manifested some destructive and omnipotent features which required individual treatment. Eventually a remission of the psychosomatic disease occurred in Riccardo and Elisa, while in Daniele's case (a baby affected from birth by a recurrent form of eczema), a diagnosis of psoriasis was recently made.

The treatment also proved inadequate in the case of six mothers who did not come to check-ups after the first meeting, and who experienced my intervention in a very persecutory way. Here, treatment could only have begun after having interpreted this kind of transference. Indeed, in such cases intervention could be said to be contraindicated, owing to the persecution it awakens. In the case of Luca, for example, his mother did not allow treatment to continue after I tried to call her attention, during the second session, to serious splitting and denial processes projected into the child. Luca was the second child of a mother affected by very serious psychiatric problems. At 3 months he developed cradle cap, which gradually receded but was replaced at 9 months by a serious form of asthmatic bronchitis, for which the baby had to be admitted to hospital. From the first meeting the mother introduced herself as an ill person in need of attention, stressing the healthiness of the child: "Luca is alright. I am the one who is not", "Luca does not stiffen when his feet are touched—rather, it's me who is afraid of hurting him when I touch him . . .", etc.

During the first consultation at 3 months, in addition to the cradle cap, the child manifested a psychogenic distal hypertonia and tremor. The next consultation did not take place until he was 10 months old, because in the meantime the mother was repeatedly admitted into the hospital psychiatric ward, where she still receives outpatient treatment. During the meeting she talked again about herself, her illness, the large number of Tavor pills she had to take. Meanwhile, the child was left alone, sitting precariously on the mattress, far from his parents. He was panting painfully. He had a rather intelligent look, but his eyes dwelt on objects in an undifferentiated way; his arms were held rigidly open and upwards; his fixed smile was striking and did not disappear from his face, even when he fell heavily on the mattress without any "parachute response". When I succeeded in calling the mother's attention to the child, she said he was very healthy, good and sociable, even though he tended to be feverish, especially at night. She said: "If he cries—which he hardly ever does—I feed him the first time, and the second time I put him to bed." At the end of the meeting I commented on Luca's behaviour, saying that it was very strange for a child to be always so good and that his painful breathing could well be his way of trying to express that there was something wrong. The father—who had remained silent and passive until that moment—seemed to be stirred, and showed interest in what I was saying. He said that it probably was so, because he had been totally absorbed in his wife's problems, which had recently been particularly difficult. Using the excuse of needing to help the child find his "parachute response", I suggested arranging a series of frequent meetings with the physiotherapist—who was present at the consultation—but so far the mother has always found excuses not to attend them.

Final considerations

I have been developing the work methodology that I have been describing in this book for about 12 years now; and I think I can conclude by saying that it has a very significant preventative function in the context of conflictual situations in danger of turning into stable pathologies. It is a technique that, while not necessarily being interpretative, seems to enable parents to use the transference situation with the specialist or the therapist. In this way parents, and particularly the mother, can achieve a deeper awareness of the problems, especially when they are able to take back into themselves projections that are affecting the child. Martha Harris (1966) believes that

> this kind of interview is one which can be conducted by workers without training in psychoanalytic psychotherapy and with varying degrees of sophistication in mental health work and concepts. . . . The essential requirement of the interviewer is, I think, a capacity to be interested in, to encompass the total situation without taking sides; to be able to encourage the parents to follow their perceptions, and to use their latent resources without increasing the feeling of helplessness, dependence and failure. Ability to refrain from giving useless advice, to distinguish between helpful advice and interference can come through bitter experience, but it can be taught and encouraged to some extent. [p. 51]

I believe that through this technique parents and children can be helped to emerge from what Cramer (1974) calls the "parasitism" of a relationship that opposes their respective processes of individuation.

CHAPTER EIGHT

The treatment and development of children with cerebral palsy

I n a work devoted to trauma due to physical handicap in children, Shirley Hoxter (1986) clearly explains the development possibilities of children affected by cerebral palsy. She states it in a very simple sentence: "The child who is affected by a physical handicap from its birth, starts life with parents being shocked by its condition, and goes on growing up in a society which also is shocked by its existence." This sentence highlights the three protagonists whose role is fundamental in the child's emotional, relational, and cognitive development—namely, the child, the parents, and the society (represented generally by the health carers).

The child

As already stated at the beginning of this book, the literature illustrates how the child's existential condition during its early life depends strictly on the functioning of its relationship with its mother, where the primitive interacting processes play an essential role in its further development. And it is clear that a serious disruption in their accomplishment must occur in the newborn who develops cerebral palsy. This is due mainly to its separation from the mother, owing to the need to keep the child in the incubator. Aguilar (1990) has stated that this condition of disruption was present in 63% of the 92 cases of cerebral palsy he has studied. In addition to this (as I have already mentioned), these children also experience intense suffering from the brain disorder (Stewart, 1985) and from the invasive medical techniques. This pain imparts to them a gloomy, sullen, complaining, unpleasant expression, making it difficult for them to experience the "aesthetic conflict" with their mother, with possible negative implications for their cognitive and emotional development. The "aesthetic conflict" has been dealt with in greater detail in chapter one.

The Barcelona school also stresses that the early disruption of the brain maturation process, occurring when the nervous system is injured, prevents an adequate containment of primitive anxieties, which is not the case with healthy newborns. Neurological paediatrics has identified several semiological elements in these patients, which define actual syndrome patterns (Touwen, 1989), such as, in particular, the hyperexcitability syndrome; the apathetic syndrome; the transient dystonic syndrome; irritability; hypo-reactivity; tremor; different types of crying; sleeping disorders; etc. A strictly neurological interpretation of symptoms is insufficient for a prognosis (as mentioned in chapter six), as clearly recognized by Touwen when he stated that of 161 newborns with such symptoms, only 10% developed cerebral palsy. This led him to conclude that "not all early symptomatology results in cerebral palsy; identical symptoms may have different prognoses. In many an infant early symptoms and signs dissolve, and development appears normal." These findings would remain without an adequate interpretation if the various violent fragmentation anxieties experienced by brain-damaged newborns were not taken into account.

During their first period of development, then, the following signs may be recognized: an elusive look, tremors, irritability, feeding and sleeping disorders, fear of having the head or feet touched and of being undressed, and other fears; postural anomalies may also be observed, such as the sudden arching in opisthotonus, or prevailing hypotonia in the trunk. From the second month onwards, these become components of a stable neuropathological pattern, which will characterize the child's cerebral palsy (Stewart, 1985). What the child needs most, particularly during this first period, is for its anxieties to be understood through experiencing someone who can help it to differentiate (Negri, 1991a).

The parents

The integration process of different parts of the self in the brain-damaged newborn is hindered not only by the violence, force, and repetitiveness of its own defence mechanisms, which are enacted in physical and sensory terms, but also by the specific emotional state of the parents, "shocked" by their child's handicap (Minde, Perrota, & Hellmann, 1988). Corominas (1983a, 1983b) and Aguilar (1983) in their work indicate that parental anxieties are already present even before the onset of the child's neurological damage, and they point out that the onset of the disorder leads to a further deterioration in their emotional state. The work in the neonatal intensive care unit made me immediately grasp the impact of these emotional experiences, which exist from the very beginning. I realized that, from the moment of birth, enormous anxiety is experienced by the parents of infants who are seriously premature or who have major neurological disorders. It is such an intense emotional state that it is difficult at first to understand to what extent it represents the parents' reaction to the traumatic birth, and to what extent it derives from concern for the child who is in danger of death or of some incapacitating chronic illness. It is therefore essential, if the child's emotional–affective dynamics are to be promoted by means of the gradual integration of its sensory skills, to consider the parents' problem first. The parents need support to cope with the anxiety deriving from the child's condition and to distinguish aspects of their own experience from that of the child's. A better understanding of violent and destructive experiences facilitates the integration processes, thereby reducing the parents' gravitation towards projective mechanisms and ultimately improving the chances of mutual individuation.

Yet the task is not easy, and I do not always succeed. Much depends on the intensity and violence of the parents' experience and on their ability to tolerate it, without immediately engaging in massive and paralysing projection dynamics. Thus the "parents' personality structure previous to the trauma" plays an important role. Anxiety may frequently be channelled into persecutory features projected into the child's paralysed limbs, thus enveloping the child in its parents' projections. When this happens, rehabilitation can take on the character of controlling the bad object, which is confined to the injured limb, to the detriment of emotional contact. The therapist who expresses his disagreement with this attitude to rehabilitation, and who works to promote separation and individuation, is regarded as hostile, as someone unable to understand the pain felt by parents with a cerebral-palsied child. It is also important to help parents to think about their feelings of guilt, which derive from such a traumatic birth. Analysing and overcoming such feelings is a very important step in the treatment. These parents tend to develop the phantasy that everything their impaired child can learn and feel depends totally on their own attitudes and behaviour: hence the risk of subjecting the child to a rigid and suffocating upbringing, which could push it unconsciously into a kind of adhesive identification.

Although, because their interaction is mutual and inextricable, it is difficult to distinguish the aspects of mentality that concern parents from those that concern the child, I would now like to consider the problems encountered by brain-damaged children which prevent their achievement of individuation.

A difficult development

The first consideration to be made in the child's treatment relates to the understanding and acceptance of the child's emotional state. As the example of Milena will show, a state of anxiety must be faced in which it seems that everything is felt as persecutory by the child. At this stage, the infant's movements play a binding role for "all its emotional experiences, which are thus held together". Given this, we can understand how the brain injury itself makes it more difficult for the child to achieve this containment and understanding of the experience: its deep anxiety is exacerbated by an irregular, uncoordinated sensori-motor function resulting from the pathology. This means that the state of emotional suffering is not conveyed to the mother in terms of a communication but is, rather, discharged violently, showing how imminently the child feels threatened by disintegration. This is why these children are usually restless, complaining, suffering, and subject to feeding and sleeping disorders; they can only be held and do not tolerate being undressed, washed, or handled; they can attain a relatively calm emotional state only when they feel closely contained, with their non-integrated parts bound together by the mother's arms.

Milena is now an intelligent 10-year-old girl. She is affected by a serious spastic quadriplegia, complicated by epileptic seizures. She is an only child, born at 31 weeks, weighing 1.320 kg. At birth she was admitted to the neonatal intensive care unit owing to respiratory distress syndrome. It was very difficult to wean her from the respirator, so she was intubated for 40 days. Already before her discharge from hospital, a hypotonia of the trunk was recorded, together with intensification of spontaneous motility and anxiety when touched on the head or dressed. During the following months, the serious neurological pattern gradually manifested itself. The physiotherapist, Antonella Fumagalli, describes the girl's first stages of development and the treatment procedures as follows:

> When discharged from the neonatal pathology ward, the baby is very irritable, averts her eyes, cries continuously, suffers from sleep disorders and anxiety when her head is touched or when she is undressed. She does not want to stay with anyone but her mother, and she, too, is very irritable. This anxiety seriously affects the physiotherapist's work. During these first months, in addition to caring for her posture, the main objective is to reassure the baby, cuddling, touching, containing and

talking to her: trying, in fact, to stimulate her to participate better in the environment and to be interested in people.

Around the fifth month, the state of anxiety has diminished slightly, and the girl starts fixing her eyes for a few moments and giving more attention to her surroundings (her mother's face while talking to her, or a noisy little toy).

Even though her mother is depressed and worried, she is very sensitive and observant of even the most imperceptible changes that occur in her child, with the help of the physiotherapist whom she meets three times a week. In this respect it is important to remember that the child's sensori-motor disorder affects not only its sensory and emotional experience, but it also impinges considerably on the mother–child tonal dialogue. It is sufficient to think, for instance, of the mutual frustration and impairment that characterize the relationship. It is therefore essential to give parents—the mother in particular—adequate support in understanding these forms of communication, which are so frustrating and difficult to accept, often marked by violent emotionality in the child.

In fact, since the child cannot find adequate means of communicating its needs, it often receives inadequate and unsuitable responses, which then aggravate its suffering. As the mother is herself seriously anxious, she may be more likely to concentrate on the physical care of the child, doing things for it, than on trying to sustain the force of its intense emotional projections.

This aspect of the problem was thoroughly analysed 12 years ago in research by Fedrizzi, Magnoni, and Cappellini (1980) on the mother–child interaction in cases of congenital quadriplegia. A relation was noted between the manner of communication between mother and child and the seriousness of the motor impairment. In the group of children with more serious verbal and gestural deficiencies, there were substantially fewer communications with the mother, as well as a use of less complex codes—both more primitive in form, and less detailed in the content of the message. A correlation between the mother–child communication and the quality of maternal behaviour and response was also found. Again this appeared both in the number of communications—which were greater when the mother had higher expectations of the child's initiative—and also in the quality of the child's messages, which were more complex when addressed to a mother of this type.

For these reasons, treatment during the first months requires the establishment of a careful, solicitous, and sensitive mode of contact by the mother and, indeed, by both parents: an attitude that could be described, as by Ferrari (1988), as "knowing what not to do to the child".

Risks involved in the first period

Considering that autism is the expression of fixations of primitive sensory attributes, it is understandable that in such situations as that of Milena, autistic mechanisms can be detected early, as a defence against intolerable anxiety. This pathology tends to select itself in a child whose sensori-motor functioning expresses itself in isolated organizational patterns of very little variation or modulation, which do not encourage integration. A barely differentiated motility such as this is not easily invested with significance and does not lend itself as a basis for thought formation. Gestures are devoid of meaning: they remain disconnected, isolated sensations and find no mental representation in symbol formation.

It is clear, then, that the child finds itself in a condition that opposes the process of integration not only as far as the motor aspect is concerned, but also with reference to the self. The major psychopathological risks for a child affected by a serious quadriplegia include not only autistic dismantling, but also a state of total non-differentiation from the object—adhesive identification and an excessive use of projective identification. The state of total identification with the object mainly occurs in children with serious brain injuries, who reject all kinds of contact apart from skin contact. And with regard to the "dismantling" condition, it is easy to see how autistic tendencies tend to be exacerbated and to become predominant in the clinical pattern.

In my experience, the risk of adhesive projection is more common. We see children of a passive demeanour who repeat, copy, adhere, but are not able to learn from experience. On the difficult road towards integration and individuation, Milena, too, resorts to adhesive identification. She refuses to be taken from her mother's arms until she is 10 months old. Later, when she allows herself to be separated, the only way of soothing her is to let her listen to nursery-rhymes (she sticks to slow, monotonous songs). When she is 18 months old, "it is difficult to know if Milena wants to do something during the session, because if you just put her on the carpet and do not soon touch her, encouraging her to do something, she just starts crying; whereas it is easier if you hold her in your arms and try to draw her attention to a toy, then wait for her to do something. . . ."

Davide, however, lives in a state of almost complete adhesive identification. He is a very beautiful 5-year-old boy with a spastic quadriplegia, complicated till the age of 4 by major epileptic seizures. His nursery-school teacher says: "He loves being held in our arms, showing no preference for any one of us; then he makes no attempt to look for objects. But if he is sat in the wheelchair or on the carpet, he does show an interest and goes to look for things; if he has a rattle, he shakes it continuously with his left hand, which he can use properly. If objects make no noise, he prefers to put them in his mouth and continuously sucks them. He goes on like this all day long." Davide has achieved satisfactory head control; he can chew and say many words; he has learned the names of his schoolmates but tends always to repeat the same name, to the teacher's surprise. From soon after his birth, once the acute phase and the serious neurological pathology were overcome, he developed a set of defence mechanisms—such as the tendency to avert his eyes and live in a condition of adhesive identification. That is why he feels at ease if he clings, either in people's arms or to an object, through the sensory experience of touching, listening, handling, or sucking.

Another risk involved in these children's development is the excessive use of projective identification. This may be clearly illustrated by the case of Alessandra. She is a first child, born prematurely at the seventh month of pregnancy and referred to me by a paediatrician. During the observation I soon notice that the little girl averts her eyes and does not smile or grasp. Her parents report that she is irritable, does not sleep, and eats without pleasure. "She is stuffed like a robot", says her father. Her motor pattern is characterized by a spastic quadriplegia. Her mother is visibly depressed, discouraged by such an unresponsive child: "You know, I always thought she was like this because she was born prematurely." However, the parents' prompt, passionate, and solicitous intervention leads to an improvement that nobody had really expected. The little girl soon starts to relate to her environment, talks, and appears intelligent and sensitive. But at the same time she prefers to spend most of her day in a phantasy world, getting her parents to play the children's' part while she plays the role of mother. If she plays with dolls, she is the physiotherapist, and the doll is Alessandra undergoing rehabilitation. It seems that the girl prefers to play the part of the adults who surround her because during the first seven months of her life she did not manage to experience an object capable of sustaining painful and intolerable projections. Now she cannot accept living like an ill and needy child. Yet this prevents her from growing up, learning, and accepting dependence. For many months, therefore, the therapist finds herself obliged to play the role of the little handicapped and messy schoolgirl, with Alessandra acting the teacher, the physiotherapist, the mother, the nurse, etc.

The problem of keeping the quadriplegic child's most disordered and needy parts integrated continues through the entire course of development. Integration requires finding a way of coexisting with the paralysed part, rather than regarding it as a dead appendix. This is very difficult to achieve, both for the child and for the people surrounding it, mainly family and health providers. Because of their own good health, they tend to be hampered by guilt when confronted with a quadriplegic child, and they are also worried by the possibility of arousing feelings of envy in the child. Hence a defensive reaction may emerge, resulting in rejection and exclusion, which take the form of admitting the child to hospital or to some other special institution. The most frequent defence, however, takes the form of idealizing certain qualities in the child—courage, intelligence, and so on—as a sort of psychological compensation for its physical vulnerability. (I have often noticed that when a quadriplegic child is integrated into a nursery or primary school, every small achievement is underlined by roaring applause from the other children, under pressure of their teacher.) The attitude of the environment can therefore collude with the child's maniacal or omnipotent aspects, which will hinder its development and prevent this child from learning from experience.

Going back to Milena's case, the physiotherapist writes:

Only around the 9th or 10th month does it become possible to organize proper physiotherapy on the carpet, without her immediately bursting out crying—provided you adopt a cautious and sweet manner. At this age the "little-hat" phobia disappears. At 16 months she still does not grasp any objects, but she makes some movement initiatives, and at home she is quieter, even though she wants to stay almost exclusively with her mother. She accepts the physiotherapy more serenely, as long as it is carried out by the physiotherapist whom she already knows, her mother is close to her, and nursery rhymes and songs are sung to her. At 18 months I can see that the child listens more carefully to what she is being told and enjoys certain parts of the story. She loves listening to fairy-tales, especially "Little Red Riding Hood". At the age of 23 months, even though her motor problem is very severe and her balance is still very fragile, Milena has considerably improved from the relational point of view. At home she no longer needs to be always held in her mother's arms; she accepts being left sitting alone for a few moments, or being held in the arms of her father or aunt. She is attentive to everything being done or said, smiling or "lalling" ("emme–au"). Her sleeping cycle becomes balanced, and she eats better. Her head control has improved; she feels more like moving; she does not crawl or roll, but, starting from a supine position, she bends forward with her head, trying to move onto her side, and starting from the prone position, she tries to push herself forward with her legs in order to crawl. She makes great efforts to grasp small toys with one hand and to bring them towards her mouth to suck them.

Although her balance is still very unstable, she accepts physiotherapy more willingly; so the sessions become more dynamic and are characterized by her active participation in play. She no longer needs nursery rhymes to reassure her; hence words can be used to describe what she is doing. She no longer cries during the physiotherapy session (which lasts three-quarters of an hour); her mother and father can remain at a certain distance, and Milena just needs to see or hear them to feel reassured. She still tends to feel anxious when nothing is actively suggested to her—when we wait for her to take the initiative in play or moving. Sudden noises or position changes still trigger the "Moro" reflex as well as crying.

The process of separation and individuation

As the physiotherapist's diary records, the therapy initially helps the mother to find the most suitable ways of supporting and handling the child in order to improve its tone and, at the same time, to enable both of them to have a more satisfactory intimate relationship. After this, the therapist concentrates mainly on the development of the mother–child relationship, trying to encourage the individuation process and facilitating separation from the mother also from a physical point of view. It is, in fact, important for the child to experience itself as physically separated from its mother and to find adequate and satisfactory postures (B. Bobath, 1967; Negri, 1982, 1983a). Living a more orderly sensori-motor experience is a way for these children "to feel helped by putting order in their mind" (Corominas, 1983b)—relinquishing the acting out of confusion through stereotypy, anarchic movement, and non-independent posture. In the treatment, therefore, which is intended to facilitate the self's individuation, the therapist pays special attention to the use of eyes, mouth, and hand. It is well known how these three components, in conjunction with a suitable postural attitude, play an important role in helping the child to individuate and differentiate. Of course what is communicated to the child through its sensory perceptions must be reinforced by the words of the therapist, helping the child give a name to things and meaning to its experience of action.

When Milena was 2 years and 6 months old, she became able to stay in the therapy room for the first time with only her father and the therapist; for the first time her mother could go out of the room for a while. On this occasion the child showed a great desire to communicate verbally with the therapist, who remarked on this. The father confirmed her observation and added that Milena had felt the urge to talk at home recently, which is why she has been "lalling" a lot.

We notice that whereas this normally happens during the first 6 to 12 months of a healthy child's development, in children affected by a severe quadriplegia it occurs around the age of 2 or 3 years. The importance of integrating the primitive sensory faculties in the brain-damaged child has already been underlined. The gradual integration of split parts of the personality promotes the formation of the self, as well as recognition of the mother's integrated image: a precise individuation and differentiation between the self and the non-self. This requires an adequate passage between introjective and projective processes, which then allows symbol formation and provides the developmental thrust towards finding increasingly more evolved forms of communication and learning.

The serious learning impairment of the severely quadriplegic child is, in my opinion, due not so much to the inadequate sensory experience, as to the defective integration of the self. This interpretation is confirmed by observations made by Stern (1985) in his analysis of how 3-week-old infants learn in relation to tactile and visual stimulants. He notes that the matching of tactile and visual experiences is made not through repeating them but, rather, on the basis of the inborn structure of the perceptive system. According to this author, no initial learning is necessary, and subsequent learning of the relation between different modes of perception is built on this inborn basic structure.

In the case of Milena, the separation and individuation process occurred at the age of 2 years and 6 months. Now counselling needs to be provided by a specialized centre so that the little girl can acquire the most effective modes of communication. The possibility of introducing Milena to nursery school is then discussed with the parents. Milena's mother immediately raises a strong objection to this latter suggestion. After some six months of reflection, during which she discusses the matter with the physiotherapist, the school staff, and myself, she agrees to try it.

This brings up the question once again of the extent to which the unconscious emotional orientation of the parents may be opposed to the process of separation and individuation.

The mothers' group

For the past three years, I have organized weekly meetings with a group of mothers, in the attempt to tackle better the problems of parents of a child with cerebral palsy, and to help them to improve their relationship with their child.

This group was started as a result of the serious depressive state of Milena's mother, Mrs G, which often led her to express her feelings about her daughter in very aggressive terms. For a long time she had complained about serious difficulties with her husband, whom she described as isolated, barely interested in and indeed irritated by the girl. Milena, too, appeared to be very depressed. She often cried; at school she was apathetic; in physiotherapy sessions she was restless and at home she showed no interest in anything. Owing to this, I had already previously suggested psychotherapy to Mrs G. She had refused and taken offence at it, telling the physiotherapist that I thought she was crazy and wanted to send her to a specialist. Yet she willingly agreed to talk with a young doctor whom she already knew and who was a trainee in my department. She attended these sessions regularly, until the doctor left the hospital. Then, together with Milena's physiotherapist— who was very worried about Mrs G—I suggested that she might take part in group therapy with other people with the same problem as hers, instead of carrying on with individual sessions.

The meetings are led by Dr Edoardo Lavelli, who works in my ward and so is already known to Mrs G. I decided to organize a group of mothers with children older than 3 years and affected by fixed patterns of cerebral palsy—the only exception being the mother of a 22-month-old twin with a very serious and irreversible motor disorder. Hour-long meetings are held once a week in the early afternoon, after which mothers go straight on to collect other children whom they may have at school. Seven or eight people participate in these meetings. After the first six months, one mother no longer participated but was still considered to be "part of the group", while another mother decided not to come after the first meeting because she regarded the problem of baby-sitting as insoluble. Apart from the external difficulties, it is important to point out that these two mothers have the greatest emotional problems of the group, and one of them in particular is affected by strongly persecutory anxieties.

Theoretical discussion
and presentation of the clinical experience

As was the case with the meetings of the group of nursing staff, the meetings with the mothers trace a group thought-movement to a point at which the group mentality can contain the emotionality of the subject under discussion. This allows the work of facilitating the child's separation and individuation to take place.

As before, four stages may be seen in the thought-movement (Vallino Macciò et al., 1990), the first being a preliminary one—the emotional atmosphere; then mourning and the representation of anxiety; recognition of the child; and hope. These stages do not follow on strictly in that order, and aspects belonging to the next stage may appear when the group is still working on the previous one. Stalemate in one of these phases prevents the thinking process from evolving and risks turning the group into a basic assumption group (Bion, 1961).

The emotional atmosphere —
the state of paranoid anxiety

For thought development to occur in the group, it is essential to be aware of the impact faced by the mothers of an emotional atmosphere full of violent and primitive experiences, often entailing a paranoid anxiety. (For further clarification of the theoretical part of the group's work see chapter two, on the work with nurses.) When anxiety reaches the level of paranoia, it may produce the disintegration of thought, thus causing paralysis of the group's functioning. The preliminary work therefore consists in setting up a group which is ready to face and work through this excessive anxiety.

In the first meetings, people often speak about intolerable and irremediable situations. As already seen in the work with nurses, a paranoid anxiety immediately appears through the group's defences; also, there is usually a member of the group who takes on the role of the thinking person, stressing his own and the other participants' ability to take stock of reality. The presence of a thinking member is useful to the leader of the group in focusing on the group's difficulties and in facing the various fears leading to irrational action. He helps to start untangling a locked situation and to allow the group to move onward, letting perceptive and attentive components emerge or re-emerge, until eventually the scope of the work to be done can be viewed.

At this preliminary stage of work, the leader confines himself to serving as a link and to identifying the fact that an intense emotional atmosphere is disturbing the accomplishment of the maternal functions. As the following example shows, the leader must be ready to be permeated by the atmosphere, letting himself be involved but not possessed by it. It may seem strange that apparently obvious functions are necessary, yet the presence of one who appears to be simply a passive listener is a necessary aspect of group dynamics. This person is, in fact, extremely active in the sense of paying attention to the group, which means that anxiety can be expressed but not acted out. In this way, paranoid anxieties are contained, and no persecutory phantasies, ethical biases, or bizarre objects (Bion, 1967a) take shape. The role of the leader is of utmost importance and sets the stage for the first reflection, through which the group can discharge the mental "toxins" of the type of anxiety that manifests itself in the form of confusion.

In the first session of this group (dated 3 April 1991), the mothers present themselves as poor victims of fate, for whom nothing goes well. They feel persecuted by malicious neighbours and relatives who also belittle their healthy children; nobody helps them. (When reading the discussions, it must be borne in mind that the people and events referred to are intended to express the thoughts and ideas of the group.) They also criticize the specialist in charge of the child's treatment, not for the treatment itself, but for marginal elements that could legitimately be criticized. The atmosphere is very persecutory and confused. The leader confines himself to expressing his understanding of the difficulties that such an ill child creates in the family environment.

This statement had the significant function of stopping the group's chaotic surge of projections and enabling the group's thinking member, Mrs T, to talk about the importance of communication. Mrs T's story was about how "people from outside" were surprised at the fact that her little girl can talk. Other participants then added their own experiences to this.

The following session has a difficult start, like all the meetings—in particular the next six, which are analysed here. Mothers find it hard to arrive on time: "Oh my God, there were so many people in the lift!" comments one lady. There is a new participant in the group, so the leader explains again what the scope and organization of the meetings is: to "compare experiences and together find solutions to the children's growth problems". Despite the difficulties of arriving on time, the group becomes very involved and keeps its link with the previous session. Mrs G demonstrates this when she says that during the previous session she had felt at ease, since "it is right to help each other, because we mothers are the only ones who know what it is to have children like ours".

Mrs V, who arrived late because her "father gave her the car with little fuel in it", asks whether her child is really spastic. A neurologist from the Public Health Service, whom she saw with her child in connection with some documents, told her he was not. She was happy to hear that. The other mothers agree in recognizing how painful it is to be confronted with the reality of the situation.

Mrs V, again, says:

"When I hear about premature newborns, I don't know, I feel so angry, but not like others, much more than that. For example, the other day I heard about a little girl, who was born at 30 weeks, like mine [besides her, in the group there are two more mothers whose children were born at 30 weeks]. Why are there so many problems, why so many preterm newborns?" The newcomer says: "No, when my little girl was in the neonatal intensive care unit, there were other healthy preterm newborns; there were only two or three unfortunate mothers like me."

Mrs G adds:

"In spite of everything, I am positive, I continue to hope."

The group's thought movement at this point has reached the moment of looking at and confronting the baby; and two main issues are dealt with: anxieties about death, and feelings of guilt.

Mourning
and the representation of anxiety

The group's anxieties about death are communicated through the story of a mother who died while giving birth to her brain-damaged child, who also died a few months later. After being discharged from the hospital where he was born, with a very unfavourable prognosis, this child was admitted to our neonatal intensive care unit, where he was taken care of by his grandparents until his death. In this way the mothers communicate that their group—which is seen as a ward—knows how to take care of children, even though they are bound to die, and through which they are able to get in touch with the experience of death. This is seen to concern not only the child but also the mother, in whom the maternal part is identified.

There is great emotional involvement and empathy with this story; but the group is pressurized by such anxiety that a sense of guilt emerges. The atmosphere of intense pain evoked by the dead mother and child is then broken by Mrs V, who says: "If I had only paid more attention to that pain . . . now things might be different." The emerging sense of guilt is so intense that it can no longer be tolerated; it stirs feelings of anger and aggressiveness towards the children which increases the sense of guilt. First Mrs V, then other mothers tell how they get angry and behave badly with their child. We see how the handicapped child, which often stimulates aggressiveness, is for its parents the projection of a deadly part of themselves—the source of an anxiety that is intolerable, and so often denied, resulting also in the child being rejected.

At this point, the leader confines himself to stressing how, during the day, one is exposed to extremely different feelings, and that sometimes under the pressure of tiredness, pessimism, and intense emotion one is no longer able to see clearly one's own state of mind or to judge the child's behaviour objectively. This comment of the leader immediately stimulates a response from Mrs T. She talks again about the story of the dead child, saying that she knows his grandparents; she then goes on talking about the maternal function of her mother-in-law in relation to her husband and herself. This function seemed to cease when their brain-damaged daughter was born: "My mother-in-law fell into a state of depression because of this, but she has now recovered." So even though the maternal function is not yet known within the group—is far away and confined to grandparents—the idea is now present and enables the group to consider vital aspects of their experience.

The mothers, in fact, dwell on the characteristics and the role of husbands, other children, and, more generally, of other members of the family.

Hope

The group has now reached a point where the real work can be begun. The various difficulties are discussed in concrete terms. The question of school is tackled and opens optimistically.

Some mothers report how this year, unlike previous ones, their children have felt welcome in the school environment "and performed better". One wonders whether this warmer welcome at school bears some relation to the mothers' group work.

Mrs T, in particular, describes a very interesting episode. The previous year, on the first day of school, the new support teacher who came from a distant town was introduced to her daughter. The teacher, without even looking at the mother, took the little girl into her arms, and the child immediately started crying. She could not be stopped, so the teacher asked the mother to leave, otherwise the girl would not have stopped crying. The mother felt very humiliated and discouraged by the teacher's attitude. Throughout the school year her daughter did not want to go to the nursery school on the days when this particular teacher was present. Mrs G knows the teacher too, because she used to work in Milena's nursery school. She confirms the teacher's inadequate attitude, recounting how she was also rejected by two brain-damaged twins who had been assigned to her.

Through this example, Mrs T expresses understanding of the significance of the maternal function in the development of the brain-damaged child: the importance of not competing with this function, and also the significance of the mother not being taken into consideration.

The atmosphere has become less persecutory, as shown by the mothers' recognition that they often tend to take up persecutory attitudes, which they define as "complaints"—as happened during the first meeting—though a mother promptly adds that even "the mothers of healthy children complain". They can now tackle their aggressiveness: "Sometimes mothers are bad. . . . I am too, sometimes I reproach Milena too much. . . . Sometimes I really could not stand it any longer, especially when Milena did not sleep at night. Once I was so exasperated that I opened the window, and I was almost about to throw her out of it, when I imagined I heard the voice of my father—who has recently died—and he said: 'What are you doing?'" She pauses, then continues, saying that she has gone through some very difficult moments. Here the leader points out that it is very important to be aware of one's difficulties and aggressive feelings towards one's children. Mrs G answers: "It's true when one is tired and alone, but fortunately my daughter now gets along well with her father, who takes care of her much more."

Mrs G's associations here are very important, since they clarify the significance of the paternal function, as something that introduces boundaries and space for reflection at times when anxiety could become overwhelming and could lead to irreparable actions. She demonstrates the twofold nature of the paternal function: the internal aspect—the father's voice, which helped her to understand and contain her exasperation at the child's demanding needs—and the external aspect, namely the actual presence of her husband, who now helps her in looking after the girl: "Since Milena started getting along well with her father, things have improved."

Recognition of the child and separation

The group now talks about children and aspects of their development: their individuality and need for autonomy, even though the process of separation is difficult to achieve. Mrs T says: "It's true, if I am patient with her, then she, too, calms down; whereas if I am nervous, she goes on crying." Mrs G says that when she left Milena alone with the physiotherapist for the second time, she went into town, and had the distinct impression that there was a cow-shed smell.

The problem under discussion proves to be so intensely emotionally involving that at one point the group move away into talk about the weather, summer, and what they will be doing during the holidays. Then they return to the separation issue, which again stirs anxieties about death and feelings of persecution. This appears when at the end of the session a mother projects this experience into an acquaintance: she reports that her neighbour once told her, "I don't know how long your daughter will live; one of my niece's daughters has died after a few years. . . . I really can't forget her!" Another mother recounts a similar episode: an aunt, whom she was visiting at a home for the elderly, said to her: "What about your daughter? Who knows whether she will survive or not; why don't you bring her here sometimes?" The mother concludes emphatically: "Far from doing that, I won't ever take her there, and I won't go and see my aunt again either—people can be horrible at times." Thus it can be seen how persecutory feelings are never resolved entirely, but reappear periodically during the sessions.

At the next session, the weather is bad, and the group participants arrive very late. They resume the issue of the paternal function, then again that of aggressiveness, and finally, at the end of the session, that of loneliness. In the following meetings they review matters already discussed and bring up new ones. The problem of the birth of the brain-damaged child is tackled anew and more thoroughly. Thus Mrs T says that recently, after a long time, she has found the courage to take her daughter to the neonatal pathology ward, since she wanted to see the place where she had been "as a baby". Noticing the worried look of the other mothers, Mrs T adds that it had not been that difficult, partly because her Delia is not seriously handicapped (she has a mild diplegia). Mrs G says that she has not yet been able to do that, but she would think about it and probably go back there.

It is interesting to note the underlying solidarity that takes shape within the group at this point: Mrs T tries not to hurt the other participants with her story of her courageous initiative in revisiting the neonatal pathology department, and the other mothers do not feel envious of this, owing to the fact that her child is the one least impaired.

Now the group is able to commit itself to reflecting on the most suitable ways to understand children with such serious communication disorders. This stage in the work is very important, because it shows a new consideration of the children themselves, who are no longer seen as a part of the parents. Before this, when I had stressed in consultations the importance of children enriching their means of communication, I had met with little response from the parents. They had answered that this effort was not necessary, because they could already understand everything their children expressed. Now, in contrast, the solution to this problem does not seem so simple. "We are not always able to understand them, especially when they are unhappy or naughty; we don't understand what they are trying to communicate, or what they want at that moment."

This issue continues to be debated during the next three sessions, in which a progressive understanding evolves, along with a new awareness of their own maternal part. This is no longer envisaged as being in a mortally affected condition—as was represented by the mother who died in childbirth—nor is it identified at one remove, as in the grandparents who help mothers with their daily cares; rather, it is to be found in that part of themselves which is able to recognize the child's qualities, needs, and desires. This is a part that is finally, after many years, felt as being vital and able to generate a healthy child. Mrs G, who has only had Milena, says: "The other day a friend of mine came to see me with her daughter. At one point she asked me, 'please, will you hold her for ten minutes?' I held her, and she told my husband: 'You see, she'd feel like having another one!' But he answered: 'Just see!' There's no question—we have talked about it, but he says that if we had another child, we would neglect Milena."

Conclusions

The group work, which is still going on, has achieved the results indicated below; and the periodical visits of the child have reflected a change in atmosphere.

In general, the atmosphere is undoubtedly less charged with projections; and in most cases an emotional contact has been established between parents and child, with a better organization of thoughts and emotions within the family, in consequence. This background allows a true work group to be established in the consulting room, comprising the parents, the physiotherapist, and myself (Vallino Macciò, 1992). As Pagliarani Zanetta writes (1990): "It is beneficial for the child to feel that a true collaborative climate and a thrust towards harmony and integration exist between the staff and all the significant people involved. This is the emotional outcome in the child's mind of attention focussed on the whole" (p. 90).

This beneficial outcome is noteworthy especially in the most serious case, that of Mrs G, which had partly motivated me to start the sessions in the first place. In recent consultations, Milena has been more involved and attentive, and she keeps looking at me throughout the examination, whereas before she hardly glanced at me except on arriving or leaving. She enjoys the elementary school and is learning well, to the satisfaction of her teachers. Her attention skills have improved. Her mother's general state of health has improved notably, with a mitigation of major symptoms such as headache, hypertension, obesity. Mrs G appears more stable and serene and has re-established a happier relationship with her partner. For almost a year she and her husband have brought Milena to consultations together. At the last check-up she told me how things have changed since the year before—when she stayed at home near the telephone when Milena was at school, always fearing they would call to inform her Milena had had one of her epileptic seizures. Now she goes out shopping or to the coffee-bar in the mornings, free from her caring commitments. She smiles while telling me all this and seems content with the new state of things.

Comparing similarities and differences in their experiences has helped the mothers to acquire a greater awareness and attentiveness both to their children's rights and to their own: avoiding collapse into states of useless resignation or sterile anger. Despite a degree of more-or-less unconscious competitiveness, the group has developed an overall solidarity in its approach, as can be seen in the clinical material. This feeling shows clearly in the warm welcome given to a newcomer (with one of the mothers accompanying her to her car), or in the anxious waiting for the return of a mother who had to leave the group for various reasons. During their daily lives, also, some mothers meet and help each other to solve the many practical problems relating to the care of their children.

We are now working towards involving the fathers more in the work, and the leader has asked the group of mothers for their opinion about the possible participation of fathers in the meetings. At first they were surprised, then they admitted a certain curiosity about the group on the part of their partners: "My husband once asked me . . . he said: 'who knows what you can talk about—you enjoy chatting' . . . he said: 'it's alright with me, as long as you don't talk about me'."

Yet the group felt that the inclusion of fathers was still premature, partly because of difficulties relating to distance or work shifts (with some working far from home). This emerged also via the story of a girl who was having difficulties at school because her teacher insisted that she finish her work within the time-span of an hour-glass, whereas she needed more time to do her work properly. This child seemed to represent the group of mothers who need more time to communicate their experiences fully, so they find the leader's proposal to be limiting, like the teacher's hour-glass.

It seemed significant, however, that at some point all the mothers, smiling or even laughing, overtly admitted their husbands' jealousy about the group meetings. As a result, most of them have invited their partners to participate in at least one group meeting, in order to let them see directly what was being discussed. In this way the fathers' interest in their wives and children comes out and also their interest in the problem in general.

In conclusion, therefore, the material of the first eight sessions is sufficient to illustrate the clinical experience: how the work develops from, in the first place, helping the participants to project less, thus allowing them to get in touch with the more painful and destructive parts of their personality. During the following sessions the work group goes through the stages described in this chapter, which are similar to those observed in relation to the staff of the neonatal intensive care unit (see chapter two; see also Negri, 1990), and to the paediatric staff involved in the care of children with AIDS (Negri, 1991b). The participants are faced with chaotic and persecutory experiences generated by the emotional atmosphere, which block out consideration of the child. Only after working through this experience and that of the next stage—mourning and the metabolism of anxiety—will mothers be able to think about the vital and hopeful aspects of themselves, their children, and their family in general. Through this they will, in particular, achieve a better separation and individuation between themselves and their children. And eventually they will be able to think about the specific needs of their children in the light of their individual characteristics and potential. This awareness allows a fleeting glimmer of hope for the future to shine through.

The health providers' group

The complexity of the pathology of cerebral palsy and the seriousness of the condition of the child with a severe quadriplegia requires an integrated overall approach by many specialists. Yet this is not easy to organize, primarily for two reasons. (1) The differing roles and knowledge of the various people means that the more a person concentrates on carrying out his work in the best and most responsible way, the more he tends to privilege his own sphere of competence. Each person's autonomy is, of course, important, but in focusing narrowly on one's own field, the overall view tends to become lost. (2) There is the problem of the deep anxiety that fills the therapist, faced with the need to sustain parents' often massive and violent projections and at the same time to work with such handicapped children.

It is very difficult to "know what not to do to the child", and not to do it: to be able to wait and observe, in order to understand its communications better and to respect its rhythms of development. It is difficult to accept the child's slow and incomplete progress, which entails being confronted continuously with one's personal feelings of impotence.

Hence the acting out of defence processes, which can lead the therapist unconsciously to use technique in an inadequate and defensive way. Moreover, it may also happen that one or more health providers in the group, coming up against their own internal inadequacy in coping with the complexity of the child's situation, blame another colleague in the group for doing a bad job. This colleague becomes the scapegoat for the unsatisfactory results of the therapy. This leads to a situation that was very common about 20 years ago, when the motor rehabilitation treatment was regarded as the most important factor for the child's recovery. Then, if the slowness or stalemate in the patient's progress became intolerable to the infant neuropsychiatrist or the physiotherapist, he might blame the failure of the therapy on the parents, for not doing enough work at home and making the child do enough physical exercise.

In a very good article, Maria Pagliarani Zanetta (1990) describes the threats to which the work group is exposed owing to its individual and group anxieties. For this reason it is important for the group leader to be aware of this phenomenon and to know when to intervene in such a way as not to interrupt the group's functioning but actually to promote its harmonization. He should encourage all its aspects to find a voice, guiding the exchange of information and communications, while being aware that the expression of personal experiences and of inter-personal disagreements must not be simply dismissed as disturbances to be eliminated, but, rather, considered as signs that—if carefully assessed—could lead to a better understanding of what is happening, and thus enable adequate solutions to be found.

In the case of the quadriplegic child, whose development depends on being able to integrate parts of its self, it is essential that there should be a parallel integration amongst the different "parts" (members) of the work-group of carers who surround it. Only in the context of the mutual awareness and integration of its carers can the child's own integration progress.

REFERENCES AND BIBLIOGRAPHY

Aguilar, J. (1983). Psicoterapie brevi nel bambino con paralisi cerebrale infantile. *Quaderni di psicoterapia infantile, Vol. 8.* Rome: Borla.

Aguilar, J., & Sariol, M. (1990). The Mother of the Child with Cerebral Palsy in the Light of the EMBU Factors. In: M. Papini, A. Pasquinelli, & E. A. Gidoni (Eds.), *Development, Handicap, Rehabilitation: Practice and Theory* (pp. 219–227). Amsterdam/New York/Oxford: Excerpta Medica, International Congress Series 902.

Als, H. (1986). A Synactive Model of Neonatal Behavioral Organization: Framework for the Assessment and Support of the Neuro-behavioral Development of the Premature Infant and His Parents in the Environment of the Neonatal Intensive Care Unit. In: J. K. Sweeney (Ed.), *The High-Risk Newborn: Developmental Therapy Perspectives. Physical & Occupational Therapy in Pediatrics.* Binghamton, NY: Haworth Press.

Amiel-Tison, C., & Dube, R. (1985). Signification des anomalies neuro-motrices transitoires. Correlations avec les difficultiés de l'âge scolaire. *Annales de Pédiatrie, 32* (1): 55–61.

Amiel-Tison, C., & Grenier, A. (1980). *Neurological Evaluation of the Newborn and the Infant.* New York: Masson.

Ammaniti, M., & Dazzi, N. (Eds.) (1990). *Affetti: Natura e sviluppo delle relazioni interpersonali.* Naples: Biblioteca di Cultura Moderna.

Anderson, G., Marks, E., & Wahlberg, V. (1986). Kangaroo Care for Premature Infants. *American Journal of Nursing, 86:* 907.

Antonacci, P. (1990). L'osservazione nel reparto di terapia intensiva neonatale di Treviglio: un approccio al neonato a rischio e ai suoi genitori. Dissertation. Regione dell'Umbria U.S.S.L., No. 3.

Aylward, G. P. (1981). The Developmental Course of Behavioural States in Preterm Infants: A Descriptive Study. *Child Development, 52:* 564–568.

Badalamenti, M., Bonarrio, P., Canziani, F., & Mangano, S. (1986). Studio epidemiologico clinico sulle paralisi cerebrali infantili in Sicilia. In: *Encefalopatie non evolutive* (pp. 23-29). Siracusa: Il Macrofago Ediprint.

Barnett, C. R., Leiderman, P. H., Grobstein, R., & Klaus, M. (1970). Neonatal Separation: The Maternal Side of Interactional Deprivation. *Pediatrics, 45* (2): 197–205.

Bender, H. (1981). Experiences in Running a Staff Group. *Journal of Child Psychotherapy, 7:* 152–157.

Benedetti, P. (1984). La nascita pretermine. *Atti XI Congresso Nazionale Società Italiana di Neuropsichiatria Infantile.*

Benedetti, P., Curatolo, P., & Galletti, F. (1978). *Il bambino con instabilità psicomotoria.* Rome: Il Pensiero Scientifico.

Benedetti, P., Ottaviano, S., Galletti, F. & Gagliasso, A. (1982). *Elementi di neurologia del primo anno di vita.* Rome: Il Pensiero Scientifico.

Benfield, D. G., Leib, S. A., & Reuter, J. (1976). Grief Response of Parents after Referral of the Critically Ill Newborn to a Regional Centre. *The New England Journal of Medicine, 294* (8): 975–978.

Berges, J., Lezine, I., Harrison, A., & Boisselier, F. (1969). Le syndrome de l'ancien prématuré, recherche sur sa signification. *Revue de Neuropsychiatrie Infantile, 17* (11): 719–777.

Bergstrom, K., & Bille B. (1978). Computed Tomography of the Brain in Children with Minimal Brain Damage: Preliminary Study of 46 Children. *Neuropädiatrie, 9:* 378–384.

Bergstrom, K., Bille, B., & Rasmussen, F. (1984). Computed Tomography of the Brain in Children with Minor Neurodevelopmental Disorders. *Neuropediatrics, 15*: 115–119.

Bernbaum, J. C., Pereira, G. R., Watkins, J. B., & Peckham, G. J. (1983). Nonnutritive Sucking During Gavage Feeding Enhances Growth and Maturation in Premature Infants. *Pediatrics, 71* (1): 41–45.

Berrini, M. E., & Carati, M. (1977). Le prime settimane di vita all'interno di una incubatrice. *Neuropsichiatria Infantile, 195*: 921–949.

Berrini, M. E., & Carati, M. (1982). L'ascolto delle madri in un reparto di maternità. *Neuropsichiatria Infantile, 246–247*: 37–50.

Bertini, M., Antonioli, M., & Gambi, D. (1978). Intrauterine Mechanisms of Synchronization: In Search of the First Dialogue. *Totus Homo, 10* (8): 73–91.

Bertolini, M., Bozzo, G., Gallo, P., Mangioni, C., Mariani, S., Nardin, E., Neri, F., Paganoni, P., Roncaglia, N., Rumi, V., & Vergani, P. (1988). Le rythme sommeil–veille du foetus. *Psychiatrie de l'enfant, 31* (1): 279–290.

Bess, F. H., Peek, B. F., & Chapman, J. J. (1979). Further Observations on Noise Levels in Infant Incubators. *Pediatrics, 63*: 100–106.

Bick, E. (1964). Notes on Infant Observation in Psychoanalytic Training. *International Journal of Psycho-Analysis, 45*: 558–566.

Bick, E. (1968). The Experience of the Skin in Early Object-relation. *International Journal of Psycho-Analysis, 49*: 484–486.

Bion, W. R. (1961). *Experiences in Groups*. London: Tavistock.

Bion, W. R. (1962). *Learning from Experience*. London: Heinemann. [Reprinted London: Karnac Books, 1984.]

Bion, W. R. (1967a). *Second Thoughts*. London: Heinemann. [Reprinted London: Karnac Books, 1984.]

Bion, W. R. (1967b). Notes on Memory and Desire. *The Psychoanalytic Forum, 2* (3). [Also in: *Cogitations* (new extended ed.). London: Karnac Books, 1992.]

Bion, W. R. (1970). *Attention and Interpretation*. London: Tavistock. [Reprinted London: Karnac Books, 1984.]

Bion, W. R. (1975–81). *A Memoir of the Future*. London: Karnac Books, 1991.

Bion, W. R. (1978). *Four Discussions with W. R. Bion*. Perthshire: Clunie Press. Also in: *Clinical Seminars and Other Works*. London: Karnac Books, 1994.

Bion, W. R. (1979). *The Dawn of Oblivion*. In: *A Memoir of the Future*. London: Karnac Books, 1991.

Bion Talamo, P. (1989). Sui gruppi "non terapeutici": L'uso del compito come difesa contro le ansie. Unpublished manuscript. Versione Rivista del Lavoro Letto Al C.R.G. di Palermo, 5 May 1989.

Bobath, B. (1967). The Very Early Treatment of Cerebral Palsy. *Developmental Medicine and Child Neurology 9* (4): 373–390.

Bobath, B. (1971a). *Abnormal Postural Reflex Activity Caused by Brain Lesion*. London: Heinemann Medical.

Bobath, B. (1971b). Motor Development, Its Effect on General Development and Application to Treatment of Cerebral Palsy. *Physiotherapy* (November).

Bobath, B., & Bobath, K. (1979). *Students' Papers* (pp. 75–107). London: The Bobath Centre.

Bobath, K. (1980). *A Neurophysiological Basis of the Treatment of Cerebral Palsy*. London: Heinemann Medical.

Bobath, K., & Bobath, B. (1964). The Facilitation of Normal Postural Reactions and Movements in the Treatment of Cerebral Palsy. *Physiotherapy* (August): 3–19.

Bollea, G. (1964). Semeiotica neurologica della prima infanzia: esame neurologico. In: P. Introzzi, *Trattato Italiano di Medicina Interna-Malattie del sistema nervoso, Vol. I* (pp. 424–439). Florence/Rome: Sadea Sansoni.

Bonassi, E., Gandione, M., Rigardetto, R., & Di Cagno, L. (1989). Il bambino prematuro che si affaccia alla vita: resoconto di tre esperienze d'osservazione. *Giornale di Neuropsichiatria dell'Età Evolutiva, 9* (3): 217–231.

Bondonio, L. (1981). Criteri metodologici del follow up e della riabilitazione precoce del neonato a rischio. *Giornale di Neuropsichiatria dell'Età Evolutiva, 1*: 7–16.

Bowlby, J. (1958). Nature of a Child's Tie to His Mother. *International Journal of Psycho-Analysis, 39*: 350–373.

Brazelton, T. B. (1973). *Neonatal Behavioral Assessment Scale*. Spastics International Medical Publications. London: Heinemann Medical.

Brazelton, T. B. (1981). *On Becoming a Family. The Growth of Attachment.* New York: Delacorte Press, Dell.

Brazelton, T. B. (1984). *Neonatal Behavioral Assessment Scale.* Lavenham, Suffolk: Lavenham Press.

Brazelton, T. B., Tronick, E., Adamson, L., Als, H., & Wise, S. (1975). Early Mother–Infant Reciprocity. *CIBA Foundation Symposium, 33* (133): 154.

Brescia, M. C. (1990). L'osservazione del bambino pretermine: la mia formazione nel reparto di terapia intensiva di Treviglio. Dissertation. Regione dell'Umbria U.S.S.L., No 3.

Brody, S. (1956). *Patterns of Mothering.* New York: International Universities Press.

Broussard, E. R., & Martner, M. S. S. (1970). Maternal Perception of the Neonate as Related to Development. *Child Psychiatry and Human Development, 1:* 17.

Brutti, C. (1975). L'osservazione del bambino come fondamento della formazione psicologica degli operatori. In: *Il bambino non visto.* Rome: Riuniti.

Bu'Lock, F., Woolridge, H. W., & Baum, J. D. (1990). Development of Coordination of Sucking, Swallowing and Breathing: Ultrasound Study of Term and Preterm Infants. *Developmental Medicine and Child Neurology, 32:* 669–678.

Burns, G. A., Deddish, R. B., Burns, W. J., & Hatcher, R. P. (1983). Use of Oscillating Waterbeds and Rhythmic Sounds for Premature Infant Stimulation. *Developmental Psychology, 19:* 746–752.

Carini, R., & Finzi, I. (1987). *Aborto volontario ripetuto e desiderio di gravidanza.* Milan: Franco Angeli.

Cioni, G., & Prechtl, H. F. R. (1988). Development of Posture and Motility in Preterm Infants. In: C. von Euler, H. Forssberg, & H. Lagercrantz (Eds.), *Neurobiology of Early Infant Behaviour.* New York: Stockton Press.

Cioni, G., Milianti, B., Castellacci, A. M., & Biagioni, E. (1988). Lo sviluppo della motricità fetale. *Atti IX Convegno di Neurologia dell'Età Evolutiva.* Rome, 15–17 April.

Clements, S. D. (1966). *Minimal Brain Dysfunction in Children.* Monograph No. 3. Public Health Service Publications, No. 1415 (New York).

Collin, M. F., Halsey, C. L., & Anderson, C. L. (1991). Emerging

Developmental Sequelae in the Normal Extremely Low Birth Weight Infant. *Paediatrics, 88* (1) (July): 115–120.

Corominas, J. (1983a). Handicap psichico: applicazioni della psicoanalisi alla psicoterapia dell'handicap. *Quaderni di Psicoterapia Infantile, Vol. 8.* Rome: Borla.

Corominas, J. (1983b). Utilizzazione di conoscenze psicoanalitiche in un centro per bambini affetti da paralisi cerebrale. *Quaderni di Psicoterapia Infantile, Vol. 8.* Rome: Borla.

Couchard, M., De Bethmann, O., Sciot, C. (1982). Interet de l'echographie cérébrale transfontanellaire iterative chez le nouveau-né de très petit poids (pp. 165–166). In: *Naissance du cerveau.* Paris: Nestlé-Guigoz.

Cramer, B. (1974). Interventions therapeutiques brèves avec parents et enfants. *Psichiatrie Enfant, 17* (1): 53–117.

De Caro, B., Orzalesi, M., & Pola, M. (1986). The Working Group as an Approach for the Psychological and Relational Training of the Personnel in a Neonatal Intensive Care Unit. *Rivista Italiana di Pediatria, 12* (5): 527–532.

De Casper, A. J., & Fifer, W. P. (1980). Of Human Bonding: Newborns Prefer Their Mothers' Voices. *Science, 208:* 1174–1176.

De Negri, M. (1990). *Neuropsichiatria Infantile.* Padua: Piccin.

Del Carlo Giannini, G. (1982). Un'ipotesi su "la vita psichica" del feto. In: *Motricità e vita psichica del feto* (pp. 104–112). Rome: Ed. Internaz. Gruppo Ed. Medico.

Di Cagno, L. (1982). L'osservazione e la conoscenza del bisogno. *Atti del Congresso* (pp. 674–694). Relazione al X Congresso Nazionale della Società Italiana di Neuropsichiatria Infantile. Sorrento, 14–17 October 1982.

Di Cagno, L. (1990). Introduzione al Convegno Dal Nascere al Divenire nella realtà e nella fantasia. *Atti Convegno Internazionale Dal nascere al divenire nella realtà e nell'infanzia* (pp. 3–11). Turin, 4–5 March. Turin: Edizioni Minerva Medica.

Di Cagno, L., & Ravetto, F. (1982). Ipotesi per un dibattito sulla malattia psicosomatica in età evolutiva. *Giornale di Neuropsichiatria dell'Età Evolutiva, 2* (1): 45–48.

Di Cagno, L., Lazzarini, A., Rissone, A., & Randaccio, S. (1984). *Il neonato e il suo mondo relazionale.* Rome: Borla.

Di Cagno, L., Peloso, A., Gruppi, E., Ferrario, M. R., & Bruno, M. (1988). Il follow up del neonato a rischio per sofferenza cerebrale. *Atti degli Incontri Internazionali multidisciplinari sullo sviluppo* (pp. 247–256). Turin, 23–24 September, 1988. Turin: CMS.

Dreyfus-Brisac, C. (1968). Sleep Ontogenesis in Early Human Prematurity from 24 to 27 Weeks of Conceptional Age. *Developmental Psychobiology*, 1: 162–169.

Dreyfus-Brisac, C. (1970). Ontogenesis of Sleep in Human Premature after 32 Weeks of Conceptional Age. *Developmental Psychobiology*, 3: 91–97.

Drillien, C. M. (1972). Abnormal Neurologic Signs in the First Year of Life in Low Birth Weight Infants. Possible Prognostic Significance. *Developmental Medicine and Child Neurology*, 14: 575.

Druon, C. (1989). L'aide au bebé et à ses parents en réanimation neonatale. *Devenir*, 1–4: 47–64.

DSM IIIR (1987). *Diagnostic and Statistical Manual of Mental Disorders* (3rd ed., revised). Washington, DC: The American Psychiatric Association.

Dubowitz, L., & Dubowitz, V. (1981). *The Neurological Assessment of the Preterm and Full-term Newborn Infant. Clinics in Developmental Medicine, No. 79.* Lavenham, Suffolk: Spastics International Medical Publications, Lavenham Press.

Dunn, J. (1980). Individual Differences in Temperament. In: M. Rutter (Ed.), *Scientific Foundations of Developmental Psychology*. London: Heinemann.

Earnshaw, A. (1981). Action Consultancy. In: Hospital Care of the Newborn: Some Aspects of Personal Stress. *Journal of Child Psychotherapy*, 7: 149–152.

Egan, D. F., Illingworth, R. S., & MacKeith, R. C. (1969). *Developmental Screening 0–5 Years. Clinics in Developmental Medicine, No. 30.* Lavenham. Suffolk: Spastics International Medical Publications, The Lavenham Press.

Elkan, J. (1981). Talking About the Birth. In: Hospital Care of the Newborn: Some Aspects of Personal Stress. *Journal of Child Psychotherapy*, 7.

Ellenberg, J. H., & Nelson, K. B. (1988). Cluster of Perinatal Events Identifying Infants at High Risk for Death or Disability. *The Journal of Pediatrics*, 113: 546–552.

Emde, R. N. (1988). Development Terminable and Interminable. *International Journal of Psycho-Analysis*, 69 (23): 25–42.

Faienza, C. (1984). Strutturazione dei cicli circadiani nel primo anno di vita. *Atti XI Congresso Nazionale Società Italiana di Neuropsichiatria Infantile.*

Faienza, C., & Capone, C. (1993). Ritmi biologici come organizzatori dello sviluppo. Milan, 18 February. Unpublished manuscript.

Fau M. (1973). La lien mère–enfant et l'avenir du prématuré. *Pediatrie, 28*: 572–574.

Fava Vizziello, G., Zorzi, C., & Bottos, M. (1992). *Figli delle macchine.* Milan: Masson.

Fazzi, E., Lanzi, G., Piazza, F., Melosi, D., Ometto, A., & Rondini, G. (1987). Lo sviluppo neuropsichico del bambino di peso alla nascita inferiore o uguale a mille grammi: studio longitudinale. *Neonatologia, 4*: 338–344.

Fedrizzi, E., Magnoni, L., & Cappellini, D. (1980). L'interazione madre–bambino nella tetraplegia congenita: relazione tra modalità di comunicazione gestuale e verbale, gravità della compromissione motoria e qualità delle condotte materne. *Neuropsichiatria Infantile, 227*: 563–592.

Ferrari, A. (1988). Paralisi cerebrale infantile: problemi manifesti e problemi nascosti. *Giornale Italiano di Medicina Riabilitativa, 3* (3): 166–170.

Ferrari, F. (1980). Aspetti clinici della sofferenza neurologica nel prematuro. *La Pediatria Medica e Chirurgica [Medical and Surgical Pediatrics], 2*: 131–138.

Ferrari, F. (1984). L'osservazione comportamentale del neonato sano e malato: la scala di Brazelton. In: M. Bertolini (Ed.), *Atti del Congresso "La nascita psicologica e le sue premesse neurobiologiche"* (pp. 313–323). Rome: IES Mercury.

Ferrari, F., Cappella, L., & Pinelli, M. (1980). Aspetti del comportamento del grande prematuro nel corso del primo semestre di vita: note preliminari. *Atti del 2. Convegno di Neurologia Neonatale.* Modena, 29–30 March.

Ferrari, F., Sturloni, N., & Cavazzuti, G. B. (1984). La maturazione dell'attività bioelettrica e dei parametri neurofisiologici che definiscono le fasi di sonno nel feto a nel neonato. In: Mario Bertolini (Ed.), *Atti del Congresso "La nascita psicologica e le sue premesse neurobiologiche".* Rome: IES Mercury.

Field, T., Ignatoff, E., Stringer, S., Brennan, J., Greenberg, R.,

Widmayer, S., & Anderson, G. (1982). Non Nutritive Sucking during Tube Feedings: Effects on Preterm Neonates in an Intensive Care Unit. *Pediatrics, 70* (3): 381–384.

Field, T., Schanberg, S. M., Scafidi, F., Bauer, C. R., Vega-Lahr, N., Garcia, R., Nystrom, J., & Kuhn, C. M. (1986). Tactile/ Kinesthetic Stimulation Effects on Preterm Neonates. *Pediatrics, 77* (5): 654–658.

Fornari, F. (1966). *La vita affettiva originaria del bambino.* Milan: Feltrinelli.

Fornari, F., Frontori, C., & Riva Crugnola, C. (1985). *Psicoanalisi in ospedale. Nascita e affetto nell'istituzione.* Milan: Raffaello Cortina.

Freud, S. (1925). *Inhibitions, Symptoms and Anxiety. S.E., 20.*

Freud, W. E. (1981). To Be in Touch. In: Hospital Care of the Newborn: Some Aspects of Personal Stress. *Journal of Child Psychotherapy, 7*: 141–143.

Gaddini, E. (1981). Note sul problema mente–corpo. *Rivista di Psicoanalisi, 26* (1): 3–29.

Gaddini, R. (1980). Patologia psicosomatica come difetto maturativo. *Rivista di Psicoanalisi, 26* (3): 381–386.

Garcia Coll, C. (1990). Behavioral Responsivity in Preterm Infants. *Clinics in Perinatoloqy, 17* (1): 113–123.

Gasparoni, M. C., Auriemma, A., Poggiani, G., Polito, E., Serafini, G., & Colombo, A. (1990). Il dolore nel neonato. *Atti del convegno.* Relazione III. Convegno di Neonatologia della Società Italiana di Pediatria. Zingonia, 26–27 January.

Giannotti, A., Lanza, A. M., & Del Pidio, F. (1984). Genesi della patologia psicosomatica, ipotesi sul ruolo svolto dalle fantasie inconsce. *Atti del Congresso* (pp. 183–191). Relazione all'XI Congresso Nazionale della Società Italiana di Neuropsichiatria Infantile. Urbino, 3–6 October.

Golberg, S., & Di Vitto, B. (1983). *Born Too Soon.* San Francisco, CA: W. H. Freeman.

Gorski, P. A., Huntington, L., & Lewkowicz, D. J. (1990). Handling Preterm Infants in Hospitals: Stimulating Controversy about Timing of Stimulation. *Clinics in Perinatology, 17* (1): 103–113.

Gottfried, A. W., & Gaiter, J. L. (1985). *Infant Stress under Intensive Care.* Baltimore, MD: University Park Press.

Gottlieb, G. (1971). Ontogenesis of Sensory Function in Birds and Mammals. In: E. Tobach, L. R. Aronson, & E. Shaw (Eds.), *The Biopsychology of Development* (pp. 67–128). New York: Academic Press.

Gottlieb, G. (1976). Conceptions of Prenatal Development: Behavioral Embryology. *Psychological Review, 83*: 215–234.

Greenacre, P. (1958). Toward an Understanding of the Physical Nucleus of Some Defence Reactions. *International Journal of Psycho-Analysis, 391*: 69–76.

Grisoni Colli, A. (1968). *L'assistenza educativa al bambino con paralisi cerebrale nella prima infanzia.* Bologna: Cappelli.

Guareschi-Cazzullo, A. (1980). Microorganicità: turbe neuropsicologiche e psicodinamiche. *Gaslini, 12* (1): 33–42.

Guareschi-Cazzullo, A. (1991). Dai disturbi generalizzati a quelli specifici dello sviluppo. *Giornale di Neuropsichiatria dell'Età Evolutiva, 11* (2): 87–94.

Haag, G. (1985). Alarmes et interventions dans les souffrances précoces. In: *Acte du Carrefour Naissances.* (November): 119–125. Ecole des parents et des éducateurs de la région toulousaine.

Haag, G. (1988). Réflexions sur quelques jonctions psycho-toniques et psycho-motrices dans la première année de la vie. *Neuropsychiatrie de l'enfance et de l'adolescence, 1*: 1–9.

Hadders-Algra, M., Touwen, B. C. L, Olinga, A. A., & Huisjés, H. J. (1985). Minor Neurological Dysfunction and Behavioural Development. A Report from the Groningen Perinatal Project. *Early Human Development, 11*: 221–229.

Hafez, E. S. E. (1975). *The Behaviour of Domestic Animals.* London: Ballière Tindal & Cassel.

Hagberg, B. (1989). Nosology and Classification of Cerebral Palsy. In: AA.VV. Le Paralisi Cerebrali Infantili. Storia Naturale delle Sindromi Spastiche. *Giornale di Neuropsichiatria dell'Età Evolutiva, 3*: 12–17.

Hagberg, B., & Hagberg, G. (1993). The Origins of Cerebral Palsy. In: T. J. David-Churchill (Ed.), *Recent Advances in Paediatrics, Vol. 11* (pp. 67–83). Edinburgh/London: Livingstone.

Hagberg, B., Hagberg, G., & Olow, I. (1984). The Changing Panorama of Cerebral Palsy in Sweden. IV. Epidemiological Trends, 1959–1978. *Acta Paediatrica Scandinavica, 73* (4): 433–440.

Hagberg, B., Hagberg, G., & Zatterstrom, R. (1989). Decreasing Perinatal Mortality. Increase in Cerebral Palsy Morbility? *Acta Paediatrica Scandinavica, 78* (2): 664–670.

Hagberg, B., Hagberg, G., Olow, I., & Von Wendt, L. (1989). The Changing Panorama of Cerebral Palsy in Sweden. V. The Birth Year Period, 1979–1992. *Acta Paediatrica Scandinavica, 78* (2): 283–290.

Hagberg, G. (1989). The Epidemiology of Cerebral Palsy in Sweden through 40 years. In: AA.VV. Le Paralisi Cerebrali Infantili. Storia Naturale delle Sindromi Spastiche. *Giornale di Neuropsichiatria dell'Età Evolutiva, Suppl., 3*: 18–24.

Harris, M. (1966). Therapeutic Consultations. In: *Collected Papers of Martha Harris and Esther Bick* (pp. 38–52). Perthshire: Clunie Press, 1987.

Harris, M. (1970). Some Notes on Maternal Containment, in: "Good Enough Mothering". In: *Collected Papers of Martha Harris and Esther Bick* (pp. 141–163). Perthshire: Clunie Press, 1987.

Harris, M. (1975). *Thinking about Infants and Young Children.* Perthshire: Clunie Press.

Harris, M. (1976). The Contribution of Observation of Mother–Infant Interaction and Development to the Equipment of a Psychoanalyst or Psychoanalytic Psychotherapist. In: *Collected Papers of Martha Harris and Esther Bick* (pp. 225–239). Perthshire: Clunie Press, 1987.

Harris, M. (1978). The Individual in the Group: On Learning to Work with the Psycho-Analytical Method. In: *Collected Papers of Martha Harris and Esther Bick* (pp. 322–339). Perthshire: Clunie Press, 1987.

Harris, M. (1979). L'apport de l'observation de l'interaction mère-enfant à la formation du psychanalyste. *Nouvelle Revue de Psychanalyse, 19.*

Harris, M. (1980). L'Autismo. *Quaderni di Psicoterapia Infantile, Vol. 3.* Rome: Borla.

Hatcher, R. (1977). The Neurophysiological Examination of the Premature Infant. *Acta Medica Auxologica, 9*: 95.

Honegger Fresco, G. (1987). *Il neonato, con amore.* Milan: Ferro.

Houzel, D. (1989). Penser les bébés; réflexions sur l'observation des nourrissons. *Revue de Médecine Psychosomatique, 19*: 27–38.

Houzel, D., & Bastard, A. (1988). Traitement à domicile en psychiatrie du nourrisson. In: B. Cramer (Ed.), *Psychiatrie du Bébé* (pp. 101–117). Paris/Geneva: Eshel.

Hoxter, S. (1986). The Significance of Trauma in the Difficulties Encountered by Physically Disabled Children. *Journal of Child Psychotherapy, 12* (1): 87–102.

Illingworth, R. S. (1966). The Diagnosis of Cerebral Palsy in the First Year of Life. *Developmental Medicine and Child Neurology, 8*: 178–194.

Imbasciati, A., & Calorio, D. (1981). *Il protomentale: psicoanalisi dello sviluppo cognitivo nel primo anno del bambino*. Turin: Boringhieri.

Isaacs, S. (1948). The Nature and Function of Phantasy. *International Journal of Psycho-Analysis, 29*: 73–97.

Ive-Kropf, V., Negroni, G., & Nordio, S. (1976). Influenza della separazione madre–bambino nel periodo neonatale sullo sviluppo di atteggiamenti materni (attaccamento). *Rivista Italaliana di Pediatria, 2*: 299–305.

Johnson, P., & Salisbury, D. M. (1975). Breathing and Sucking during Feeding in the Newborn. *CIBA Foundation Symposium, 33* (119): 135.

Jouvet, M. (1978) Does a Genetic Programming of the Brain Occur during Paradoxical Sleep? In: P. A. Buser & A. Rougeul-Buser (Eds.), *Cerebral Correlates of Conscious Experience*. Amsterdam: North-Holland.

Kaplan, D. M., & Mason, E. A. (1960). Maternal reactions to premature birth viewed as an acute emotional disorder. *American Journal of Orthopsychiatry, 30*: 539–552.

Kellerhals, J., & Pasini, W. (1977). *Perche l'aborto?* Milan: Mondadori.

Kennell, J. H., Slyter, H., & Klaus, M. H. (1970). The Mourning Response of Parents to the Death of a Newborn Infant. *The New England Journal of Medicine, 283* (7): 344–349.

Kennell, J. H., Trause, M. A., & Klaus, M. H. (1975). Evidence for a Sensitive Period in the Human Mother. *CIBA Foundation Symposium, 33*: 87–101.

Kennell, M., Klaus, M. H., McGrath, M. D., Robertson, D., & Hinkley, D. (1991). Continous Emotional Support During Labor in a US Hospital. A Randomized Controlled Trial. *Journal of the American Medical Association, 265* (17): 2197–2201.

Kestemberg, E. (1977). *Le devenir de la prematurité*. Paris: Presses Universitaires de France.

Klaus, M. H., & Kennell, J. H. (1970). Mothers Separated from Their Newborn Infants. *Pediatric Clinics of North America, 17*: 1015–1037.

Klaus, M. H., & Kennell, J. H. (1971). Care of the Mother of the High-Risk Infant. *Clinical Obstetrics and Gynecology, 14*: 926.

Klaus, M. H., & Kennell, J. H. (1983a). *Bonding: The Beginnings of Parent–Infant Attachment*. New York/Scarborough, Ontario: New American Library; Mosby.

Klaus, M. H., & Kennell, J. H. (1983b). Risultati ottenibili con interventi nei reparti per prematuri. *Clinica Pediatrica del Nord America, 15* (3): 866.

Klaus, M. H., Kennell, J. H., Robertson, S., & Sosa, S. S. (1980). Effects of Social Support during Parturition on Maternal and Infant Morbidity. *British Medical Journal, 295* (8 September): 585–587.

Klaus, M. H., Kennell, J. H., Geraud, N., & McAlpine, I. (1972). Maternal Attachment. Importance of the First Post-Partum Days. *New England Journal of Medicine, 286*: 460.

Klein, M. (1946). Notes on Some Schizoid Mechanisms. *International Journal of Psycho-Analysis, 27*: 99–110.

Klein, M. (1952a). On Observing the Behaviour of Young Infants. In: M. Klein, P. Heimann, S. Isaacs, & J. Riviere, *Developments in Psychoanalysis*. London: Hogarth Press. [Reprinted London: Karnac Books & The Institute of Psychoanalysis, 1989.]

Klein, M. (1952b). Some Theoretical Conclusion Regarding the Emotional Life of the Infant. In: M. Klein, P. Heimann, S. Isaacs, & J. Riviere, *Developments in Psychoanalysis*. London: Hogarth Press. [Reprinted London: Karnac Books & The Institute of Psychoanalysis, 1989.]

Klein, M. (1955). On Identification. In: *New Directions in Psychoanalysis*. London: Tavistock. [Reprinted London: Karnac Books, 1985.]

Klein, M., & Stern, L. (1971). Low Birth Weight and the Battered Child Syndrome. *American Journal of Diseases of Children, 122* (July): 15–18.

Knobloch, H., & Pasaminick, B. (1959). Syndrome of Minimal Cerebral Damage in Infancy. *Journal of the American Medical Association, 170*: 1384.

Korner, A. F. (1986). The Use of Waterbeds in the Care of Preterm Infants. *Journal of Perinatology, 6* (2): 142–147.

Korner, A. F. (1989). Infant Stimulation: The Pros and Cons in Historical Perspective. *Zero to Three* (December): 11–17.

Korner, A. F. (1990). Infant Stimulation Issues of Theory and Research. *Clinics in Perinatology, 17* (March, No. 1): 173–184.

Korner, A. F., Brown, B. V., Dimiceli, S., Forrest, T., Stevenson, D. K., Lane, N. M., Costantinou, J., & Thom V. A. (1989). Stable Individual Differences in Developmentally Changing Preterm Infants: A Replicated Study. *Child Development, 60*: 502–513.

Korner, A. F., Brown, B. V., Reade, E. P., Stevenson, D. K., Fernbach, S. A., & Thom, V. A. (1988). State Behavior of Preterm Infants as a Function of Development, Individual and Sex Differences. *Infant Behavior and Development, 11*: 111–124.

Korner, A. F., Guilleminault, C., Van den Hoed, J., & Baldwin, R. B. (1978). Reduction of Sleep Apnea and Bradycardia in Preterm Infants on Oscillating Waterbeds: A Controlled Polygraphic Study. *Pediatrics, 61*: 528–533.

Korner, A. F., Kraemer, H. C., Haffner, M. E., Cosper, L. M. (1975). Effects of Waterbed Flotation on Premature Infants: A Pilot Study. *Pediatrics, 56* (3): 361–367.

Korner, A. F., Kraemer, H. C., Reade, E. P., Forrest, T., Dimiceli, S., & Thom, V. A. (1987). A Methodological Approach to Developing an Assessment Procedure for Testing the Neurobehavioral Maturity of Preterm Infants. *Child Development, 58*: 1478–1487.

Korner, A. F., Lane, N. M., Berry, K. L., Rho, J. N., & Brown, B. V. (1989). Sleep Enhanced and Irritability Reduced in Preterm Infants: Differential Efficacy of Three Types of Waterbeds. *World Association for Infant Psychiatry and Allied Disciplines. Fourth Congress.* Lugano, Switzerland, 20–24 September.

Korner, A. F., Schneider, P., & Forrest, T. (1983). Effects of Vestibular–Proprioceptive Stimulation on the Neurobehavioral Development of Preterm Infants: A Pilot Study. *Neuropediatrics, 14*: 170–175.

Korner, A. F., & Thoman, E. B. (1970). Visual Alertness in Neonates as Evoked by Maternal Care. *Journal of Experimental Child Psychology, 10*: 67–78.

Kramer, L. I., & Pierpoint, M. S. (1976). Rocking Waterbeds and Auditory Stimuli to Enhance Growth of Preterm Infants. *The Journal of Pediatrics, 88*: 297–299.

Kreisler, L. (1981). *L'enfant du dèsordre psychosomatique.* Private publication.

Kreisler, L., Fain, M., & Soulé, M. (1967). La clinique psycho-somatique de l'enfant. Les états frontières dans la nosologie. *La Psychiatrie de l'Enfant, 10*: 157–198.

Kreisler, L., & Soulé, M. (1985). L'enfant prematuré. In: S. Lebovici, R., Diatkine, & M. Soulé (Eds.), *Traité de Psychiatrie de l'Enfant et de l'Adolescence.* Paris: Masson.

Lamour, M., & Lebovici, S. (1991). Les interactions du nourrisson avec ses partenaires: evaluation et modes d'abord préventifs et thérapeutiques. *La Psychiatrie de l'Enfant, 34* (1): 171–275.

Lax, R. F. (1972). Some Aspects of the Interaction Between Mother and Impaired Child: Mother's Narcissistic Trauma. *International Journal of Psycho-Analysis, 53*: 339.

Lebovici, S. (1978). La contribution de la psychanalyse des enfants à la connaissance et à l'action sur les jeunes enfants et les familles déprimées. *Communication Congrès. int. de Psychoanal. d'Enfants.* Unpublished.

Lebovici, S. (1983). *Le nourrisson, la mère et le psychanalyste* (p. 377). Paris: Centurion, Paidos.

Leiderman, P. H., Leifer, A. D., Seashore, M. J., Barnett, C. R., & Grobstein, R. (1973). Mother–Infant Interaction: Effects of Early Deprivation, Prior Experience and Sex of Infant. *Early Development, 51*: 154–175.

Leiderman, P. H., & Seashore, M. J. (1974). Mother–Infant neonatal Separation: Some Delayed Consequences. In: *CIBA Foundation Symposium, 33. Parent–Infant Interaction* (pp. 213–232). Amsterdam: Association of Scientific Publishers.

Le Métayer, M. (1989). Bilan neuromoteur (cérébromoteur) du jeune enfant. *Encyclopédie Médico Chirurgicale* (Paris), *26028* (B20-4): 1–26.

Lester, B. M., Boukydis, C. F. Z., McGrath, M., Censullo, M., Zahr, L., & Brazelton, T. B. (1990). Behavioral and Psychophysiologic Assessment of the Preterm Infant. *Clinics in Perinatology, 17* (1): 155–171.

Le Vagerese, L. (Ed.). (1983). Un enfant, prematurement. *Les Cahiers du nouveau, Vol. 6.* Paris: Stock.

Lezine, I. (1977). La futura sorte dell'ex prematuro. In: *Le devenir de la prematurité*. Paris: Presses Universitaires de France.

Lombardi, F., & Argese, M. G. (1982). Problematiche psicologiche delle madri di bambini in incubatrice. *Neuropsichiatria Infantile, 246-247*: 51-66.

Long, J. G., Lucey, J. F., & Philip, A. G. S. (1980). Noise and Hypoxemia in the Intensive Care Nursery. *Pediatrics, 65*: 143-145.

Long, J. G., Philip, A. G. S., & Lucey J. F. (1980). Excessive Handling as a Cause of Hypoxemia. *Pediatrics, 65*: 203-207.

Lussana, P. (1984). Con Mrs. Bick discutendo l'osservazione madre–bebé accanto alle varianti dell'interazione analista–analizzando. *Rivista di psicoanalisi, 3*: 356-367.

Maestro, S., Marcheschi, M., Muratori, F., & Tancredi, R. (1989). Comprensione e nosografia delle psicosi precoci, un contributo metodologico. *Giornale di Neuropsichiatria dell'Età Evolutiva, 9* (4): 305-314.

Magagna, J. (1987). Three Years of Infant Observation with Mrs. Bick. *Journal of Child Psychotherapy, 13* (1).

Male, P., Doumic-Girard, A., Benhamon, F., & Schott, M. C. (1975). *Psychothérapie du premier age*. Paris: Presses Universitaires de France.

Mancia, M. (1980). *Neurofisiologia e vita mentale*. Bologna: Zanichelli.

Marazzini, P. M., & Mazzucchelli, S. (1990). Supporto e sostegno ai genitori del neonato pretermine in terapia intensiva: modulazione della comunicazione. *Giornale di Neuropsichiatria dell'Età Evolutiva, 10* (4): 357-363.

Marcheschi, M., Pfanner, P., & Masi, G. (1989). *La clinica dei disturbi di apprendimento*. Rome: Borla.

Marshall, R. E., & Kasman, C. (1980). Burnout in the Neonatal Intensive Care Unit. *Pediatrics, 65*: 1161-1165.

Martin, R. J., Herrell, N., & Rubin, D. (1979). Effect of supine and prone position on arterial oxygen tension in the preterm infant. *Pediatrics, 63*: 528-531.

Mautner, H. (1959). *Mental Retardation. Its Care, Treatment and Physiological Base* (p. 30). New York: Pergamon Press.

McFarlane, A. (1975). Olfaction in the Development of Social Preferences in the Human Neonate. *CIBA Foundation Symposium: Parent–Infant Interaction, 33*: 103-117.

McGee, R., Williams, S., & Feehan, M. (1992). Attention Deficit Disorder and Age of Onset of Problem Behaviors. *Journal of Abnormal Child Psychology, 20* (5): 487–502.

McGraw, M. B. (1946). Maturation of Behavior. In: L. Carmichael (Ed.), *Manual of Child Psychology*. New York: John Wiley.

McGrath, P. J. (1987). An Assessment of Children's Pain: A Review of Behavioral, Psychological and Direct Scaling Techniques. *Pain, 31*: 147.

Meier, P., & Anderson, G. C. (1987). Responses of Small Preterm Infants to Bottle and Breast-Feeding. *American Journal of Maternal and Child Nursing, 12*: 97–105.

Meltzer, D. (1980). L'autismo. *Quaderni di Psicoterapia Infantile, Vol. 3*. Rome: Borla.

Meltzer, D. (1986). *Studies in Extended Metapsychology*. Perthshire: Clunie Press.

Meltzer, D. (1992). *The Claustrum*. Perthshire: Clunie Press.

Meltzer, D., Bremner, J., Hoxter, S., Weddell, D., & Wittemberg, I. (1975). *Explorations in Autism: A Psychoanalytical Study*. Perthshire: Clunie Press.

Meltzer, D., & Harris, M. (1983). *Child, Family and Community: A Psycho-Analytical Model of the Learning Process*. Paris: Organization for Economic Co-operation and Development.

Meltzer, D., & Harris, M. (1985). La fiaba dello sviluppo infantile. *Giornale di Neuropsichiatria dell'Età Evolutiva, 5* (3): 275–283.

Meltzer, D., & Harris Williams, M. (1988). *The Apprehension of Beauty*. Perthshire: Clunie Press.

Michaelis, R., Parmelee, A. H., Stern, E., & Haber, A. (1972). Activity States in Premature and Term Infants. *Developmental Psychobiology, 6*: 209–215.

Milani Comparetti, A. (1982a). Protagonismo e identità dell'essere umano nel processo ontogenetico. In: A. Ianniruberto, F. A. Catizone, & L. Bovicelli (Eds.), *Giornate italo–americane di ultrasonografia* (pp. 202–212). Bologna: Monduzzi.

Milani Comparetti, A. (1982b). Semeiotica neuroevolutiva. *Prospettive in Pediatria, 48* (10–12): 305–314.

Milani Comparetti, A., & Gidoni, E. A. (1976). Dalla parte del neonato: proposte per una competenza prognostica. *Neuropsichiatria Infantile, 173*: 5–17.

Miller, A. J. (1982). Deglutition. *Physiological Review, 62*: 129–183.

Mills, J. N. (1975). Development of circadian rhythms in infancy. *Chronobiologia*, 2: 363–371.

Minde, K., Perrotta, M., & Hellmann, J. (1988). Impact of Delayed Development in Premature Infant on Mother–Infant Interaction: A Prospective Investigation. *The Journal of Pediatrics*, *112* (1): 136–142.

Minde, K., Shosenberg B., Marton P., Thompson, J., Ripley, J., & Burns, S. (1980). Self-help Groups in a Premature Nursery: A Controlled Evaluation. *The Journal of Pediatrics*, *96*: 933–940.

Minde, K., Trehub S., Corter C., Boukydis, C., Celhoffer, L., & Marton, P. (1978). Mother–Child Relationships in the Premature Nursery: An Observational Study. *Pediatrics*, *61*: 373–379.

Moceri, A., & Pagnin, A. (1983). Bambini in incubatrice: analisi catamnestica di un gruppo di soggetti portati in consultazione. *Giornale di Neuropsichiatia dell'Età Evolutiva*, *3* (1): 37–46.

Negri, R. (1973). La metodica dell'osservazione come approccio psicodinamico al bambino. *Neuropsichiatria Infantile*, *149–150* (November–December): 879–906.

Negri, R. (1980). Problemi metodologici della prevenzione del neonato a rischio. *Neuropsichiatria Infantile*, *230–231*: 859–878.

Negri, R. (1982). L'evoluzione della teoria Bobathiana nel trattamento del bambino con paralisi cerebrale infantile. *Giornale di Neuropsichiatria dell'Età Evolutiva*, *2* (3): 299–307.

Negri, R. (1983a). Fisioterapie e rieducazioni precoci alla luce dei problemi dello sviluppo emotivo. *Quaderni di Psicoterapia Infantile*, *8*: 82–98. Rome: Borla.

Negri, R. (1983b). Introduzione al dibattito: il neonato in neuropsichiatria infantile. *Giornale di Neuropsichiatria dell'Età Evolutiva*, *3* (1): 59–70.

Negri, R. (1984). Segni predittivi di schizofrenia infantile nel primo anno di vita. In: C. L. Cazzullo (Ed.), *La schizofrenia in età evolutiva, fattori di rischio e predittività* (pp. 45–52). Rome: Il Pensiero Scientifico.

Negri, R. (1985). La disfunzione cerebrale minima (MBD) ed il neonato ad alto rischio. *Giornale di Neuropsichiatria Infantile*, *4* (4): 363–375.

Negri, R. (1986). Riconoscimento e cura della psicosi nei primi mesi di vita. *Psichiatria dell'infanzia e dell'adolescenza, 6*: 673–684.

Negri, R. (1988). Una metodologia di intervento sui genitori del neonato gravemente pretermine all'interno del reparto di terapia intensiva. *Giornale di Neuropsichiatria dell'Età Evolutiva, 8* (3): 225–239.

Negri, R. (1989a). La fiaba della nascita del fratello nello sviluppo emotivo. *Quaderni di Psicoterpia Infantile, Vol. 18* (pp. 45–75). Rome: Borla.

Negri, R. (1989b). L'osservazione del neonato: metodologia di studio dei processi mentali. *Quaderni di Psicoterapia Infantile, Vol. 18* (pp. 100–116). Rome: Borla.

Negri, R. (1989c). Problematiche di psicosomatica nei primi mesi: una proposta di intervento. *Quaderni di Psicoterapia Infantile, Vol. 19* (pp. 217–231). Rome: Borla.

Negri, R. (1990). Il gruppo di lavoro con le infermiere di un reparto di patologia intensiva neonatale. *Atti Convegno Internazionale dal nascere al divenire nella realtà e nella fantasia* (pp. 251–256). Turin, 4–5 March. Turin: Minerva Medica.

Negri, R. (1991a). Il ruolo delle dinamiche emotivo–affettive nella comunicazione e nell'apprendimento del bambino con grave tetraplegia. *Saggi, 17* (1): 13–20.

Negri, R. (1991b). L'istituzione ospedaliera e il bambino con AIDS: il problema della formazione psicologica degli operatori. *Psichiatria dell'infanzia e dell'adolescenza, 58*: 227–238.

Negri, R. (1992). La prevention neuro-psychologique chez les nouveau-nées gravement prématurés (< 1,000 gr). In: J. P. Relier (Ed.), *Progrés en Neonatologie, Vol. 12* (pp. 263–290). Paris: Karger.

Negri, R., Boccardi, G., Nissim, S., Pagliarani, M., & Vallino Macciò, D. (1990). Il gruppo in patologia intensiva: osservare a "porte aperte" il neonato pretermine. *Quaderni di Psicoterapia Infantile, Vol. 22* (pp. 137–147). Rome: Borla.

Negri, R., Guareschi Cazzullo, A., Vergani, P., Mariani, S., & Roncaglia, N. (1990). Correlazione tra vita prenatale e formazione della personalità. Studio preliminare attraverso l'osservazione di due gemelli. *Quaderni di psicoterapia infantile, Vol. 22* (pp. 148–165). Rome: Borla.

Orzalesi, M., Maffei, G., De Caro, B., & Pellegrini-Caliumi, G. (1989). Il dolore nel neonato. *Prospettive in Pediatria, 76*: 295–302.

Pagliarani Zanetta, M. (1990). Globalità e persona. *Rivista Italiana di Psicoterapia e Psicosomatica, 2* (3): 77–93.

Paine, R. S. (1960). Neurologic Examination of Infants and Children. *Pediatric Clinics of North America, 4*: 471–510.

Paine, R. S. (1962). Minimal Chronic Brain Syndromes in Children. *Developmental Medicine and Child Neurology, 4*: 21–27.

Paine, R. S., Brazelton, T. B., Donovan, D. E., Drorbaugh, J. E., Hubbell, J. P., & Sears, E. M. (1964). Evolution of Postural Reflexes in Normal Infants and in the Presence of Chronic Brain Syndromes. *Neurology, 14*: 1036–1048.

Palacio Espasa, F., & Manzano, J. (1982). La consultation thérapeutique des trés jeunes enfants et leur mère. *La Psychiatrie de l'Enfant, 25* (1): 5–27.

Paludetto, R. (1977). The Importance of Interpersonal Interactions in Perinatal Care. *Rivista Italiana di Pediatria, 3*: 431–436.

Papousek, H., & Papousek, M. (1979). Early Ontogeny of Human Social Interaction: Its Biological Roots and Social Dimensions. In: K. Foppa, W. Lepenies, & D. Ploog (Eds.), *Human Ethology: Claims and Limits of a New Discipline* (pp. 456–489). Cambridge: Cambridge University Press.

Peiper, A. (1963). Cerebral Function in Infancy and Childhood. (Translation of: *Die Eigenart der Kindlichem Hirntätigkeit*, 3rd ed., 1961). New York: Consultants Bureau.

Peloso, A., Bruno, M., Ferrario, M. R., & Gruppi, E. (1989). Un'esperienza di lavoro con i genitori all'interno di un Centro Immaturi. *Giornale di Neuropsichiatria dell'Éta Evolutiva, 9* (March, No. 1): 59–66.

Peltzam, P., Kitterman, J. A., Ostwald, P. F., Manchester, D., & Heath, L. (1970). Effects of incubator noise on human hearing. *The Journal of Auditory Research, 10*: 335–339.

Perez Sanchez, M. (1990). *Baby Observation: Emotional Relationship during the First Year of Life*. London: Karnac Books.

Perlmen, J. M., & Volpe, J. J. (1983). Fuctioning in the Preterm Infant: Effects on Cerebral Blood Flow Velocity, Intracranial Pressure and Arterial Blood Pressure. *Pediatrics, 72*: 329–334.

Pfanner, P., Marcheschi, M., Masi, G., & Brizzolara, D. (1990). Neuropsicologia e riabilitazione dei disturbi dello sviluppo. *Giornale di Neuropsichiatria dell'Età Evolutiva, 10* (1): 27–37.

Pfanner, P., Marcheschi, M., Muratori, F., & Maestro, S. (1990). I segni precoci dell'evoluzione deficitaria nelle disarmonie evolutive. *Psichiatria dell'infanzia e dell'adolescenza, 57:* 19–26.

Pinkerton, P. (1965). The Psychosomatic Approach in Child Psychiatry. In: J. G. Howells (Ed.), *Modern Perspectives in Child Psychiatry* (pp. 306–335). London: Oliver & Boyd.

Pisaturo, C., & Ciravegna R. (1983). Criterio prognostico del danno neurologico da sofferenza feto-neonatale. *Giornale di Neuropsichiatria dell'Età Evolutiva, 3* (1): 27–36.

Porter, F. (1989). Pain in the Newborn. *Clinics in Perinatology, 16:* 549–564.

Prechtl, H. F. R. (1984). *Continuity of Neural Functions from Prenatal to Post-natal Life.* Lavenham Suffolk: Lavenham Press.

Prechtl, H. F. R., & Beintema, B. J. (1964). *A Neurological Study of Newborn Infants.* Clinics in Developmental Medicine, No. 28. London: Heinemann.

Prugh, D. (1953). Emotional problems of premature infants' parents. *Nursing Outlook, 1:* 461–464.

Regini, P., & Scavo, M. C. (1990). La care dei nati a rischio: aspetti di continuità terapeutica dall'unità di terapia intensiva neonatale al follow-up dei primi anni di vita. *Giornale di Neuropsichiatria dell'Età Evolutiva, 10* (1): 69–76.

Reid, M. (1993). Joshua—Life after Death: The Replacement Child. *Journal of Child Psychotherapy, 18* (2): 109–138.

Riva Crugnola, C. (Ed.) (1993). *Lo sviluppo affettivo del bambino.* Milan: Raffaello Cortina.

Rivarola, A. (1991). Interazione comunicativa nei primi anni di vita: modalità di osservazione e strategie di intervento. *Saggi, 17* (1): 29–35.

Robson, K. S. (1967). The Role of Eye-To-Eye Contact in Maternal Infant Attachment. *Journal of Child Psychology and Psychiatry, 8:* 13–25.

Robson, K. S., & Moss, H. A. (1970). Patterns and Determinants of Material Attachment. *Journal of Pediatrics, 77* (6): 976.

Rosenfeld, H. A. (1978). The Relationship Between Psychosomatic Symptoms and Latent Psychotic States. *The Bulletin of the British Psychoanalytical Society, 4* (April): 14–29.

Rustin, M. (1988). Encountering Primitive Anxieties: Some Aspects of Infant Observation as a Preparation for Clinical Work with Children and Families. *Journal of Child Psychotherapy, 14* (2): 15–28.

Saint-Anne Dargassies, S. (1972). Neurodevelopmental Symptoms during the First Year of Life. *Developmental Medicine and Child Neurology, 14*: 235–264.

Saint-Anne Dargassies, S. (1974). *Le développement neurologique du nouveau-né a terme et prematuré.* Paris: Masson.

Salk, L. (1973). The Role of Heartbeat in the Relation between Mother and Infant. *Scientific American, 228*: 24–29.

Salzberger-Wittenberg, I. (1990). Therapeutic Work with Parents of Infants. *Atti Convegno Internazionale Dal Nascere al Divenire nella realtà e nella fantasia* (pp. 205–221). Turin, 4–5 March. Turin: Minerva Medica.

Sameroff, A. J., & Emde, R. N. (1989). *Relationship Disturbances in Early Childhood: A Developmental Approach.* New York: Basic Books.

Sandri, R. (1991). *La maman et son bébé: un regard.* Lyon: Cesura.

Satge, P., & Soulé, M. (1976). L'accueil et la prise en charge des parents dans un centre de néonatologie. *Expansion Scientifique,* Paris.

Sauvage, D. (1984). *Autisme du nourrison et du jeune enfant (0–3 ans).* Paris: Masson.

Schaffer, R. H. (1974). Behavioural Synchrony in Infancy. *New Scientist, 62* (April): 16–18.

Schaffer, R. H. (1974). Early Social Behaviour and the Study of Reciprocity. *Bulletin of the British Psychological Society, 27*: 209–216.

Schaffer, R. H. (Ed.) (1977). *Studies in Mother–Infant Interaction.* London: Academic Press.

Schmid-Kitsikis, E. (1985). *Théorie et clinique du fonctionnement mental.* Brussels: Mardaga.

Schneider, P. B. (1968). Remarques sur les rapports de la psychanalyse avec la médecine psychosomatique. *Revue Française de Psychanalyse, 32*: 645–672.

Scott, S., Cole, T., Lucas, P., & Richards, M. (1983). Weight Gain and Movement Patterns of Very Low Birthweight Babies Nursed on Lambswool. *The Lancet, 2* (8357): 1014–1016.

Scott, S., & Martin, R. (1981). Nursing Low Birthweight Babies on Lambswool. *International Cerebral Palsy Society Bulletin* (June): 14–17.

Sheridan, M. D. (1977). *Children's Developmental Progress from Birth to Five Years: The Stycar Sequences*. Windsor, Berkshire: NFER Publishing.

Solnit, A. J., & Green, M. (1959). Psychologic Considerations in the Management of Deaths on Pediatric Hospital Services. I. The Doctor and the Child. *Family Pediatrics* (July): 106–112.

Sosa, R., Kennell, J., Klaus, M., Robertson, S., & Urrutia, J. (1980). The Effect of a Supportive Companion on Perinatal Problems, Length of Labor, and Mother–Infant Interaction. *The New England Journal of Medicine, 303* (September 11): 597–600.

Soulé M., Houzel, D., & Bollaert, S. (1976). Les psychoses infantiles précoces et leur traitement. *La Psychiatrie de l'Enfant, 19* (2): 341–397.

Sperling, M. (1953). Psychosis and Psychosomatic Illness. In: *Annual Meeting of the American Psychoanalytic Association*. Los Angeles, CA, 2 May.

Spitz, R. A. (1951). Psychogenic Diseases in Infancy. An Attempt at Their Etiologic Classification. *Psychoanalytic Study of the Child, 6*: 255–275.

Stern, D. N. (1985). *The Interpersonal World of the Infant*. New York: Basic Books.

Stewart, A. (1985). Early Prediction of Neurological Outcome When the Very Preterm Infant Is Discharged from the Intensive Care Unit. *Annales de Pédiatrie, 32* (1): 27–37.

Stork H. (1983). Le repérage précoce des psychoses infantiles et les perspectives de prévention. *Neuropsychiatrie de l'enfance et de l'adolescence* (5–6): 248–252.

Sumner, E. (1993). Pain: Its Implications in the Newborn and Premature Baby. *Abstracts* (pp. 93–96). *Relazione al Convegno "Problemi Medici e Chirurgici in Éta Pediatrica". Specialisti a confronte*. Bergamo, 15–16 October.

Szure, R. (1981). Infant in Hospital. In-hospital Care of the Newborn: Some Aspects of Personal Stress. *Journal of Child Psychotherapy, 7*: 137–159.

Tajani, E., & Ianniruberto, A. (1990). The Uncovering of Fetal

Competence. In: M. Papini, A. Pasquinelli, & B. E. A. Gidoni (Eds.), *Handicap, Rehabilitation: Practice and Theory*. Amsterdam: Excerpta Medica.

Thomas, A. (1963). *Behavioral Individuality in Early Childhood*. New York: New York University Press.

Thomas, A., & Autgaerden, S. (1966). *Locomotion from Pre- to Postnatal Life. Clinics in Developmental Medicine, No. 24*. Lavenham, Suffolk: Spastics International Medical Publications, Lavenham Press.

Torrioli, M. G. (1987). Il problema della valutazione in una consulenza in un Centro di Terapia Intensiva Neonatale. Prospettive Psicoanalitiche nel lavoro istituzionale. *Il Pensiero Scientifico*, 5 (December, No. 2): 237–244.

Touwen, B. C. L. (1989). Early Detection and Early Treatment of Cerebral Palsy: Possibilities and Fallacies. *Giornale di Neuropsichiatria dell'Età Evolutiva*, 4: 31–38.

Touwen, B. C. L. (1990). Variability and Stereotypy of Spontaneous Motility as a Predictor of Neurological Development of Preterm Infants. *Developmental Medicine and Child Neurology*, 32: 501–514.

Trevisan, C. P., De Zanche, C., Miottello, P. G., Pellegri, A., Sartor, C., Baradei, C., Pianalto, P., Deutch, F. (1986). *Epidemiologia delle paralisi cerebrali infantili nel Veneto: i tassi di incidenza 1974–83 per le province di Padova e Vicenza. Encefalopatie infantili non evolutive* (pp. 7–16). Siracusa: Il Macrofago-Ediprint.

Tronick, E. Z. (1989). Emotions and Emotional Communication in Infants. *American Psychologist* (February): 112–118.

Tronick, E. Z., Scanlon, B., & Scanlon, W. (1990). Protective Apathy, a Hypothesis About the Behavioral Organization and Its Relation to Clinical and Physiologic Status of the Preterm Infant During the Newborn Period. *Clinics in Perinatology, 17* (March, No. 1): 125–154.

Tustin, F. (1986). *Autistic Barriers in Neurotic Patients*. London: Karnac Books.

Vallino Macciò, D. (1984). Emozioni e sofferenze del bambino al primo incontro. *Conferenza tenuta presso l'Istituto di Neuropsichiatria Infantile di Milano*, 2 June. Unpublished paper.

Vallino Macciò, D. (1992). La consultazione psicoanalitica del bambino in età prescolare come applicazione dell'osservazione psicoanalitica del bambino. Conference held in Verona, 6 November. Unpublished paper.

Vallino Macciò, D., Boccardi, G., Negri, R., Nissim, S., & Pagliarani, M. (1990). Funzione del gruppo di discussione nell'osservazione del bambino in famiglia. *Quaderni di Psicoterapia Infantile*, 22: 121–136. Rome: Borla.

Viola, M. (1991). "Modi" e "ritmi" nella relazione bambino–madre. In: A. Imbasciati & L. Cena, *La vita psichica primaria*. Milan: Masson.

Vojta, V. (1974). *Die zerebralen Bevegungsstörungen im Säuglingsalter*. Stuttgart: Ferdinand Enke Verlag.

Volpe, J. J. (1987). *Neurology of the Newborn*. Philadelphia, PA: Saunders.

Volpe, J. J. (1991a). Neurologic Sequelae in the Premature Infant: Relation to Specific Types of Brain injury. *Abstract* (pp. 55–59). *15th International Symposium of Neonatal Intensive Care, San Remo (Imperia)*, November 14–17.

Volpe, J. J. (1991b). Cognitive Deficits in Premature Infants. *New England Journal of Medicine 325* (4): 276–277.

Watillon-Naveau, A. (1992). Les psychothérapies précoces mères–enfants. Unpublished paper.

Wender, P. H. (1971). *Minimal Brain Dysfunction in Children*. New York: Wiley.

White, J. L., & Labarba, R. C. (1976). The Effects of Tactile and Kinesthetic Stimulation on Neonatal Development. *Psychobiology, 6*: 569–577.

Winnicott, D. W. (1958). Primary Maternal Preoccupation. In: *Collected Papers: Through Paediatrics to Psycho-Analysis*. London: Tavistock.

Winnicott, D. W. (1965). *The Maturational Processes and the Facilitating Environment*. London: London: Hogarth. [Reprinted London: Karnac Books & The Institute of Psychoanalysis, 1990.]

Winnicott, D. W. (1966). Psychosomatic Illness in Its Positive and Negative Aspects. *International Journal of Psycho-Analysis, 47*: 510–516.

Winnicott, D. W. (1971). *Therapeutic Consultations in Child Psychiatry*. London: The Hogarth Press.

Wolff, P. H. (1966). The Causes, Controls and Organization of Behavior in the Neonate. *Psychological Issues, 5*: 1–105.

INDEX

acoustic stimulation, of infant in
  incubator, 5
active sleep, 129
"activity" of infant, 87
adhesive identification, 39, 186,
  187, 200, 203, 204
aesthetic conflict, 18–19, 38, 95,
  161, 198
affective disorder, 187
affective spasms, 172
Aguilar, J., 198, 199
AIDS, 220
alarm symptoms, in neonatal
  neurology, 158–174
Alberico [infant], 12
Alessandra [infant], 204, 205
Als, H., 7
Amiel-Tison, C., 133, 150, 176,
  177
Anderson, C. L., 115, 164
Andrea [infant], 67
Angela [nurse], 65, 72, 75
Anna [nurse], 76, 77

anorexia, 15, 170
anxiety:
  catastrophic, 35, 161, 168
    and sense of guilt, 35–37
  claustrophobic, 157–158, 170
  confusional, 161, 163
  death, 16–18, 17, 18, 38, 213
  fragmentation, 180, 181, 198
  paranoid, 54, 57, 161, 163,
    211
    of mothers of children with
    cerebral palsy, 211–213
  in neonatal intensive care
    unit, 53
  primary, 170
  primitive, 50, 160, 180, 198
  representation of, 59, 65, 210
    by mothers of children with
    cerebral palsy, 213–214
    by staff, 59–65
apathetic syndrome, 159, 198
apathy, protective, 14, 94
apnoea, 15, 100, 101, 115

archaic reflexes of infant, 137
Argese, M. G., 13
artificial ventilation, 97
aspiration syndrome, 97
asthma, 172
asthmatic bronchitis, 193
atopic dermatitis, 172
attention:
    deficit disturbance with
        hyperactivity, 176
    disorders of, 164, 175
Aurora [infant], 192
Autgaerden, S., 132, 133, 141
autism, 19, 175, 188, 192, 203
autistic moment, 118
automatic walking, of infant, 140
Aylward, G. P., 108

Badalamenti, M., 165
Bambina [nurse], 61, 72–78
Barnett, C. R., 50
Bastard, A., 164
"battered baby" syndrome, 14
Baum, J. D., 114, 115
beauty, of infant, 18, 27
behavioural disorder, 176, 180
Beintema, B. J., 109, 133
Bender, H., 50
Benedetti, P., 81, 133, 174
Benfield, D. G., 13
Benhamon, F., 164
Berges, J., 179
Berges syndrome, 180
Bergstrom, K., 177
Bernbaum, J. C., 114
Berrini, M. E., 4, 10, 29
Bess, F. H., 89
"beta-elements" [Bion], 53
Bianca [infant], 39–40
Bick, E., xiv, xvi, 45, 82, 84, 104,
        107, 180, 182
Bille, B., 177
Bion, W. R., xvi, 10, 19, 53, 54, 71,
        125, 159, 163, 210, 211
Bion Talamo, P., 45, 71
Bobath, B., 141, 158, 207

Bobath, K., 141
Boccardi, G., 52
body scheme, 6
Boisselier, F., 179
Bollaert, S., 164
Bollea, G., 133
Bonarrio, P., 165
bottle-feeding, 115, 188
Bottos, M., 162
Bowlby, J., 13, 14
"boyfriend", of infant, 109, 111
brain:
    disorder, 187, 198
    minimal damage syndrome, 173,
        176, 178
Brazelton, T. B., 3, 4, 11, 13, 109,
        133, 144, 147
breast:
    as aesthetic object, 18
    -feeding, 6, 13, 19, 63, 115, 117,
        158, 161, 162, 163
    relationship, 9, 10
    toilet-, 121–123
Brody, S., 4
bronchopneumonia, 97
Broussard, E. R., 13
Bu'Lock, F., 114, 115
"burn-out" syndrome, 43
Burns, G. A., 7

Camilla [infant], 153
Canziani, F., 165
Capone, C., 109
Cappellini, D., 202
Carati, M., 4, 11, 29
Carla [infant], 98
Carlo [infant], 62, 75
catastrophic anxiety, 35, 161, 168
    and sense of guilt, 35–37
cerebral palsy, 1, 30, 38, 159, 160,
        164, 165, 175, 177
    children with, treatment of, 197–
        228
cerebral suffering, symptom of, 3
Chapman, J. J., 89
Chiara [child], 24, 27, 31

child, *passim* (*see also* infant)
adopted, claustrophobic
    anxieties of, 158
with AIDS, 220
autistic, 19, 175, 188, 192, 203
beauty of, 18–19, 27
with cerebral palsy, 197–199
    development of, 200–228
dying, parents of, 39–41
hospitalization of, effects of, 11
living, image of in parents' mind,
    95
Cioni, G., 131, 132
circadian rhythm, 166
claustrophobic anxieties, 157–158,
    170
Clements, S. D., 175
co-ordination impairment, 175
Cole, T., 7
colic, 167, 170, 171, 172, 173, 192
Coll, G., 85
Collin, M. F., 164, 165
colon, irritable, 170
communication, disorders of, 164,
    217
conflict, aesthetic, 18–19, 38, 95,
    161, 198
confusional anxiety, 163
consciousness, state, of infant, 133
constipation, 170
containment:
    experience of, 121–123
    insufficient, 169, 180, 181, 198
    maternal, 169
continuous positive pressure
    endonasal tube, 100
Corominas, J., 92, 159, 199, 207
Couchard, M., 131
Cramer, B., 164, 195
crying, types of, 159
Curatolo, P., 174
cutaneous stimulation, of infant in
    incubator, 5

Daniele [infant, twin of Elisa], 105,
    193

Davide [infant], 204
death:
    anxiety, 16–18, 38, 213
    instinct, 77
De Bethmann, O., 131
Deddish, R. B., 7
De Caro, B., 3, 43
De Casper, A. J., 7, 89
Del Carlo Giannini, G., 159
Delia [infant], 217
Del Pidio, F., 174
De Negri, M., 174
denial:
    mother's, 173, 191
        projected into child, 193
    of own death, 27
    parents', 15
depression:
    anxiety of, 10
    of mother, 118–121
    post-partum, 19
deprivation somatic disorder, 170
development:
    of child with cerebral palsy,
        200
    disorder, 160, 164, 165–169
        specific, 176
developmental language disorder,
    177
Di Cagno, L., 169, 170
disorder (*see also* syndrome)
    affective, 187
    attention, 164, 175
    behavioural, 176, 180
    brain, 187, 198
    communication, 217
    deprivation somatic, 170
    development, 160, 164, 165–
        169
        specific, 176
    developmental language, 177
    emotional, 13
        and relational, 178
    feeding, 2, 165, 169, 172, 201
    functional, 170
    gastrointestinal, 172

disorder (*continued*)
    language
        and hearing, 175
        and speech, 175
    memory and thinking, 175
    motor, 210
    neurodevelopmental, 177
    neurological, 159, 160, 166,
        179, 199
    of perceptive functions, 185
    perinatal, 177
    psychic, 175
    psychopathological, 162
    psychosomatic, 164, 169, 170,
        172, 173, 190, 191
    psychotic, 166
    relational–cognitive, 164, 165
    respiration, 169
    sensorimotor, 202
    skin, 169
    sleep, 2, 159, 165, 169, 172,
        174, 198, 201
    somatic, 170, 171
    specific development, 174
Donatella [child], 188, 189
Donatella [physiotherapist], 72, 75
Doumic-Girard, A., 164
Downs syndrome, 55, 56, 58, 61,
    64
Dreyfus-Brisac, C., 106, 159
Drillien, C. M., 181
Dube, R., 176
Dubowitz, L., 133
Dubowitz, V., 133
Dunn, J., 3
dyspractognosies, 175
dyspraxias, 175
dystonic syndrome, 176, 177
    transient [Drillien], 159, 176,
        181, 198

Earnshaw, A., 2
echographic observation, 112,
    132
eczema, 167, 172, 192, 193
Egan, D. F., 133

electroencephalographic
    irregularities, 175
Elena [nurse], 69
Elisa [infant, twin of Daniele], 104,
    105, 193
Elisabetta [infant], 23–26, 27, 28,
    29, 30–35, 37, 54, 55, 57,
    61, 69
Elkan, J., 11
Ellenberg, J. H., 165
Emde, R. N., 87
emotional disorder, 13
    and relational disorder, 178
endotracheal tube, 30
Extremely Low Birth Weight
    Infants (ELBWI), 88

Facchetti, R., 70
Faienza, C., 109
Fain, M., 169
father, approach with, in intensive
    care unit, 13–16
Fau, M., 15
Fava Vizziello, G., 162
Fazzi, E., 164, 165
Federica [infant], 168
Federica [nurse], 55
Fedrizzi, E., 202
feeding:
    behaviour of neonate, 114
        effect of on mother, 3
    bottle-, 115, 188
    breast-, 6, 13, 19, 63, 115, 117,
        123, 158, 161, 162, 163
    child with catastrophic anxiety,
        168
    containment during, 5
    continuous, 20
    disorder, 2, 165, 168, 169, 170,
        172, 173, 198, 201
    in incubator, 15
    milk-, 114, 115
    naso-gastric, 49, 70
    naso-jejeunal, 26, 114
    passivity in, 168
    problems, 100, 168

satisfactory experience of, 161
self-, 172
tube, 44, 97, 100, 102, 103,
    104, 110, 112
Ferrari, A., 106, 203
Field, T., 7, 114
Fifer, W. P., 7, 89
follow-up after discharge, 5
foot grasp, of infant, 137
Fornari, F., 116
Francesca [infant], 161, 163
free motility, 150
Freud, S., 159, xiv, xv, xvi
Freud, W. E., 50
Fumagalli, A., 201
functional disorder, 170

Gaddini, E., 169
Gaddini, R., 169
Gagliasso, A., 133
Gaiter, J. L., 4
Galletti, F., 133, 174
Gasparoni, M. C., 3
gastric tube, 49
gastrointestinal disorder, 172
gaze aversion, 165, 168
Giacomo [infant], 29, 51, 61, 88,
    90, 93–105, 107–123, 126–
    128
Gianluca [infant], 67
Giannotti, A., 174
Gidoni, E. A., 133
Giorgio [infant], 73
Giovanna [infant], 187, 188, 189
"girlfriend", of infant, 109, 111,
    122
Giuliana [infant], 122
Giuseppe [infant], 167, 168, 189
Giusy [nurse], 65
"good-enough" mother, 10
Gorski, P. A., 85
Gottfried, A. W., 4
grasping, of neonate, 103–108
Green, M., 39
Greenacre, P., 171
Grenier, A., 133, 150, 176

Grisoni Colli, A., 133
Grobstein, R., 50
Guareschi Cazzullo, A., 45, 174
guilt, sense of, and catastrophic
    anxiety, 35–37

Haag, G., 162, 164
Hadders-Algra, M., 176
Hafez, E. S. E., 150
Hagberg, B., 164, 165
Hagberg, G., 164, 165
Halsey, C. L., 164
hand grasp, of infant, 137
Harris, M., xvi, 43, 45, 46, 66, 84,
    158, 169, 172, 184, 186,
    195, xiv
Harrison, A., 179
Harris Williams, M., xvi, xvii–xxiii,
    18, 19, 95, 161
Hatcher, R. P., 7
health providers' group, 221–228
Hellmann, J., 199
Herrell, N., 7
hiccups, 169, 172, 181
hope, generation of, 66
hospitalization, of child, effects of,
    11
Houzel, D., 82, 164
Hoxter, S., 197
Huisjés, H. J., 176
Huntington, L., 85
hyperactive syndrome, 175, 178
hyperexciteability, 159, 176, 198
hyperkinesia, 167, 175, 180, 181
hypermotility, 172
hyper-reactivity, of infant, 85
hypertonia, 172, 176
    distal, 181, 194
    plastic, 168
    psychogenic, 132
hypokinesia, 175
hypo-reactivity, 85, 159, 198
hypotonia, 166, 199, 201

Ianniruberto, A., 115, 159
idealization, 10, 76

identification
    adhesive, 39, 186, 187, 200,
        203, 204
    projective, 10, 53, 60, 71, 72,
        113, 116, 123, 203, 204
    unconscious, of nurses with
        parents and child, 72
identifications, organization of,
    162
Illingworth, R. S., 133
incorporation, of nipple, 119
individuation, 207, 208, 209, 210,
    220
    establishing, 38, 200
        and brain-damaged children,
            200, 204, 209
        and parasitism, 187, 195
    mother–infant, 118, 207–209
        early, 118, 207
    separation–, processes of, 30–
        35
infant, passim (see also child)
    first days of life of, 88–90
    importance of interaction with
        mother, 3
    irritability of, 97–99
    observation, 160–161
        difficulties of, 84
        effect of on nurses, 125
        function of, 124
        and infant care, 65–69
        methodological aspects of, 82–
            84
        and nurses' written
            descriptions, 69–71
    physiognomy of, 91–95
    psychopathological symptoms
        of, 2
    suffering of, 90–91
infantile self, mother's, 10
integration, 4, 38, 186, 191, 199,
    200, 203, 204, 205
    defective, 169, 172, 174, 186,
        208
    lacking drive for, 160
    motor, 151

non-, 172, 180
    psychosomatic, 169
    role of mother in, 162, 163, 169
    of self, 151
    of sense organs, 94, 159, 161
    of sensori-motor experiences,
        101, 113–118
    of sensory capacity, 160, 199
        lack of, 166
    of split parts of personality, 208
interaction, neonate's first signs of
    need for, 97
interrupted pregnancy, 27–30
intervention, methodology of, 20–
    27
introjection, 102, 104, 112, 113,
    116, 161, 180
    early processes of, 99–113
irritability, 2, 91, 132, 159, 165,
    166, 168, 169, 172, 185,
    198
Isaacs, S., 159
Ive-Kropf, V., 13, 14

Jacopo [infant], 34
jealousy, of elder child, 31
Johnson, P., 4, 115
Jouvet, M., 159

kangaroo care, 6
Kasman, C., 45
Kellerhals, J., 28
Kennell, J., 3, 13, 14, 15, 21, 22,
    38, 39
Kennell, M., 11
Klaus, M. H., 3, 11, 13, 14, 15, 21,
    22, 38, 39, 50
Klein, M., xiii, 14, 71, 116, 118,
    121
Knobloch, H., 177
Korner, A. F., 7, 101, 109, 131,
    133
Kreisler, L., 169, 170, 171, 179,
    180, 181

Labarba, R. C., 7

lamb's fleece, 7, 48, 89, 97, 106, 107, 127
language and hearing disorder, 175
Lanza, A. M., 174
Lavelli, E., 210
Lax, R. F., 18
learning impairment, 175
Lebovici, S., 164
Leib, S. A., 13
Leiderman, P. H., 3, 50
Lester, B. M., 85
Lewkowicz, D. J., 85
Lezine, I., 2, 179, 180
Lino [infant], 66, 67, 68, 69
"little hat" phobia, 1, 2, 132, 206
"little schoolboy", 107
Lombardi, F., 13
Long, J. G., 125
Luca [infant], 193, 194
Lucas, P., 7
Lucey, J. F., 125
Lucia [nurse], 33, 35, 36, 61, 63, 76, 77, 78
Luciana [nurse], 61, 63, 64, 65, 66, 67, 68
Lussana, P., 82

MacKeith, R. C., 133
Maffei, G., 3
Magagna, J., 82
Magnoni, L., 202
Male, P., 164
Mancia, M., 159
Mangano, S., 165
Manzano, J., 174, 187, 193
Marazzini, P. M., 15
Marco [infant], 111
Maria [infant], 17, 20, 37
Maria [nurse], 55, 56, 57, 58
Maria Gratia [nurse], 76, 77
Marshall, R. E., 45
Marta [infant], 92, 107, 127
Martin, R. J., 7, 89
Martner, M. S. S., 13
maternal attachment process, 14

maternal containment, 169
maternal self, 10
Mautner, H., 177
Mazzucchelli, S., 15
McFarlane, A., 4
McGrath, P. J., 3
Meier, P., 115
Melody [infant], 63
Meltzer, D., xiii, 18, 19, 45, 66, 95, 104, 157, 158, 159, 161, 166, 186
memory and thinking disorder, 175
merycism, 172, 173, 190
Michela [infant], 190
Milani Comparetti, A., 86, 87, 131, 132, 133
Milena [infant], 200, 201, 203, 204, 206–210, 215, 216, 218, 219
Miller, A. J., 115
Mills, J. N., 165
mimic rigidity, 167
Minde, K., 14, 15, 38, 93, 94, 199
minimal brain dysfunction syndrome, 164, 174–194
mirror resonance, 45, 52, 56, 60, 64
of nurses, 71–75
Moceri, A., 180
Monica [nurse], 66, 67, 68, 72, 73, 74, 75
Moro reflex, 137, 144, 207
Moss, H. A., 13
mother:
approach with, in intensive care unit, 13–16
depression of, 118–121, 174, 192
"good-enough", 10
good internal, 10
–infant individuation, 118
during post-partum period, 9
of premature infant, 14
presence of, near incubator, 94
visual contact with, 161–163

motility:
  free, 150
  spontaneous, 132, 144, 152,
    181, 201
  of very small infant, 89
motor:
  development, 86, 87
  disorder, 210
  integration, 151
  perceptual impairment, 175
  restlessness, 2, 169, 174, 181
mourning, 12, 174, 210, 220
  and anxiety, 59–65
    of mothers of children with
      cerebral palsy, 213–214

narcissistic wound, 18.
naso-gastric feeding, 49
  tube, 49, 70, 114
naso-jejeunal feeding, 26, 114
  tube, 49, 114
Negri, R., xiv, xvi, 1, 4, 37, 45, 52,
    59, 82, 84, 94, 158, 159,
    166, 169, 171, 173, 179,
    199, 207, 220
Negroni, G., 13
Nelson, K. B., 165
neonate, see child, infant
neurodevelopmental disorder, 177
neurological disorder, 159, 160,
    166, 179, 199
neurological screening, 133
neurology, neonatal, 158
neuropsychological evaluation, 44,
    82, 124, 128, 129, 164
  of infant, prior to discharge,
    131–149
neutral role, concept of, 59–71
newborn, see child, infant
Nordio, S., 13
nurses: see staff

object:
  differentiation, 97–99, 123
  relations, emotional experiences
    deriving from, 113–118

observation, infant:
  difficulties of, 84
  methodological aspects of, 82
  "open-door", 127
Odone, G., 16, 21
Oedipus complex, xviii, 28
Olinga, A. A., 176
Olow, I., 165
"open-door" observation of
    newborn, 5, 51, 66, 69,
    126, 127, 128
organizational patterns, child's
    first, 110–112
Orzalesi, M., 3, 45
Oscar [infant], 70–71
osteotendinous reflex responses, of
    infant, 137
Ottaviano, S., 133

Pagliarani Zanetta, M., 218, 221
Pagnin, A., 180
Paine, R. S., 133, 177, 178
Palacio Espasa, F., 174, 187, 193
Paludetto, R., 15
Papousek, H., 3
Papousek, M., 3
paranoid anxiety, 54, 57, 163
  of mothers of children with
    cerebral palsy, 211
  in neonatal intensive care unit,
    53
"paranoid mother" phenomenon,
    48, 46
parents:
  approach with, in intensive care
    unit, 13–16
  of child with cerebral palsy, 199–
    200
  empathic attitude of staff to, 48–
    49
  image of living child in mind of,
    95–96
Pasaminick, B., 177
Pasini, W., 28
Peckham, G. J., 114
Peek, B. F., 89

Peiper, A., 27, 132, 133
Pellegrini-Caliumi, G., 3
Peltzam, P., 89
perceptive functions, disorder of, 185
Pereira, G. R., 114
Perez Sanchez, M., 82
perinatal disorder, 177
Perrotta, M., 199
persecutory projection, 28
personality, two-dimensional, 180
Philip, A. G. S., 125
Piera [nurse], 55, 59, 67
Pinkerton, P., 170
Pino [infant], 15, 20–21
placing reaction, of infant, 140
Plutarch, 27
pneumothorax, 97
Pola, M., 45
Porter, F., 3
post-discharge follow-up of infant, 149–155
post-discharge treatment, 183–195
post-partum depression, 19
postural anomalies, 198
practognostic functions, development of, 179
Prechtl, H. F. R., 109, 131, 132, 133, 159
pregnancy, interrupted, 27–30
preventive environmental actions, 4, 5–6, 82–84, 93, 102, 127
primary anxiety, 170
projection, 15, 18, 28, 76, 78, 112, 113, 116, 167, 180, 184, 187, 189, 191, 195, 200, 202, 204, 205, 212, 214, 218, 221
early processes of, 104–106
projective identification, 10, 60, 71, 72, 113, 116, 123, 203, 204
beta elements discharged as, 53
propositional competence, 91, 93, 94, 95, 96, 117, 128, 132
[Milani Comparetti], 87–88

[Stern], 87
proprioceptive stimulation, 6
Prugh, D., 13
psoriasis, 193
psychic disorder, 175
"psychic skin", 162
psychopathological conditions, 157–182
psychophysical syndrome, 171
psychosis, 164, 179, 187, 189
early, 165–169
psychosomatic disorder, 164, 169–174, 190–193
psychotic disorder, 166

quadriplegia, 201, 203, 208, 221
congenital, 202
spastic, 204, 205

Rasmussen, F., 177
Ravetto, F., 169, 170
reflex:
Moro, 137
smile, 106, 112
standing, of infant, 140
tonic, symmetric and asymmetric, 137
reflexology, 132
Reid, M., 12
relational–cognitive disorder, 164, 165
respiration, disorder, 169
Reuter, J., 13
Riccardo [infant], 193
Richards, M., 7
risks, psychopathological, 157–182
Roberto [infant], 55
Robertson, S., 11
Robson, K. S., 13, 14, 161
rooting response, 137
Rosenfeld, H. A., 169, 170
Rubin, D., 7
Rustin, M., 84

Sabrina [infant], 60, 62, 63, 120, 124

safety rhythm, 117
Saint-Anne Dargassies, S., 3, 132, 133, 141
Salisbury, D. M., 4, 115
Salk, L., 89
Salzberger-Wittenberg, I., 183
Sandri, R., 82
Satge, P., 15.
Scanlon, B., 14
Scanlon, W., 14
Schaffer, R. H., 3
Schilder, P., xv
Schneider, P. B., 171
Schott, M. C., 164
Sciot, C., 131
Scott, S., 7, 89
screening, neurological, 133
Seashore, M. J., 3
self:
    infantile, mother's, 10
    maternal, 10
    -regulation of infant, 87
sensori-motor disorder, 202
sensori-motor experiences,
        integration of, 113–118
separation, 154
    anxiety of, 10
    depressive pain of, defence
        against, 111
    difficulties:
        father's role in, 191
        and psychosomatic disorders, 173
    in extubation, 110
    -individuation, 30–35, 38, 170, 200, 209, 210, 220
    of child with cerebral palsy, 207
    importance of, 154
    from infant, of nurses, 109, 111, 120, 121, 124
    of mother and child, 3, 50
        early, 19, 198
        facilitating, 207
    problems:
        of child, 187, 216–218

of mother, 174
Sheridan, M. D., 133
Silvia [infant, twin of Stefano], 104, 105
Simone [infant], 171, 172
skin, 180
    disorder, 169
    maternal function as [Bick], 179, 180
    "psychic", maternal function as [Bick], 162
    "second" [Bick], 180, 182
sleep:
    active, 129
    disorder, 2, 159, 165, 169, 172, 174, 198, 201
    of neonate, 103–108
    –waking:
        cycles, ontogenesis of, 106
        organization, 109
Slyter, H., 39
smile, reflex, 106, 112
"social fitness" of infant, 87
Solnit, A. J., 39
somatic disorder, 170, 171
Sonia [infant], 192
Sosa, R., 11
Soulé, M., 15, 164, 169, 170, 179, 180, 181
sound therapy, 5, 89, 97
specific development disorders, 174–210
Sperling, M., 169
Spitz, R. A., 170
splitting, 15, 113, 121–123, 167, 168, 170, 191
    mother's, projected into child, 193
staff:
    meeting
        example of, 54–57, 61, 63–65, 68–69, 72–76
        "open-door" observation session, 66–67
        role of leader, 57
    of neonatal intensive care unit,

working with, 43–79
work group, experiences in, 75–78
standing reflex, of infant, 140
starting, abrupt, of neonate, 103–108, 129
Stefania [infant], 28
Stefano [infant, twin of Silvia], 104
stereotypy, 160
Stern, D. N., 14, 118, 208
Stevens [infant], 61, 63, 64
Stewart, A., 198, 199
stimuli, visual and auditory, infant's response to, 137
Stork, H., 164
sucking:
    and apnoea, 115
    at breast, 119
    difficulties, 6, 49
    effective, 115
    interaction through, 93
    introjection through, 103, 116
    milk-, 115
    non-nutritional, 6, 7, 97, 114
    as pleasurable experience, 161
    rhythmic, 116
    taste stimulation for, 114
    vigorous, 68
Sumner, E., 3
Susanna [nurse], 66, 67
syndrome (see also disorder)
    apathetic, 159, 198
    aspiration, 97
    "battered baby", 14
    Berges, 179
    "burn-out", 43
    dystonic, 159, 198
    hyperactive, 178
    hyperexcitability, 198
    hyperkinetic, 175
    neurotic, 178
    psychopathic, 178
    psychophysical, 171
    psychosomatic, 169, 171, 173, 190–193

respiratory distress, 201
schizophrenic, 178
transient dystonia, 176
Szure, R., 2

Tajani, E., 115, 159
taste stimulation, 7, 89, 102, 114
    of infant in incubator, 5
thinking disorder, 175
Thomas, A., 3, 132, 133, 140, 141
Thomas static straightening reflex, 140
thorax, "stretching", 6
thought formation, 113–118
toilet–breast, 121–123
Tomsic, S., 70
tonic reflex, symmetric and asymmetric, 137
Touwen, B. C. L., 131, 132, 158, 159, 160, 176, 198
tracheal tube, 23
    removal of, 99–103
transient dystonic syndrome, 159, 198
Trause, M. A., 3
treatment, post-discharge, 183–195
tremor, 2, 159, 169, 172, 181, 190, 194, 198
Treviglio–Caravaggio (Bergamo) Hospital, 1, 13
Trevisan, C. P., 165
Tronick, E. Z., 14, 85, 94, 133
trunk tone, of infant, 140
trusting, experience of, 121–123
tube:
    endotracheal, 23, 25, 27, 30
    -feeding, 44, 97, 100, 102, 103, 104, 110, 112
    gastric, 49
    naso-gastric, 49, 114
    naso-jejeunal, 49, 114
    naso-tracheal, 44, 70
    tracheal, 23, 99
Tustin, F., 117, 158

unconscious identification, of
    nurses, with parents and
    child, 72
University of Milan, 1

Vallino Macciò, D., 45, 52, 71, 185,
    186, 210, 218
variability, of functions, 160
ventilation, artificial, 97, 99, 100
vestibular stimulation, 6
Viola, M., 116, 158
Vojta, V., 132, 133, 140, 141
Vojta position reflex, 140, 152
Volpe, J. J., 133, 164, 165
vomiting, 172
Von Wendt, L., 165

waking, first, of neonate, 108–110

water mattress, 6, 7, 71, 94, 101
Watillon-Naveau, A., 164
Watkins, J. B., 114
Wender, P. H., 178
White, J. L., 7
Williams, S., xvi
Winnicott, D. W., 9, 169, 170, 191
Wolff, P. H., 109, 133
Woolridge, H. W., 114, 115
work group, 45, 52, 56, 72, 73, 75,
    76, 78, 107, 120, 124, 125,
    185, 191, 218, 220, 222
wound, narcissistic, 18

Yuri [infant], 74

Zatterstrom, R., 165
Zorzi, C., 162